Palgrave Texts in Counselling and Psychotherapy

Series Editors

Arlene Vetere, Family Therapy and Systemic Practice, VID
Specialized University, Oslo, Norway
Rudi Dallos, Clinical Psychology, Plymouth University,
Plymouth, UK

This series introduces readers to the theory and practice of counselling and psychotherapy across a wide range of topical issues. Ideal for both trainees and practitioners, the books will appeal to anyone wishing to use counselling and psychotherapeutic skills and will be particularly relevant to workers in health, education, social work and related settings. The books in this series emphasise an integrative orientation weaving together a variety of models including, psychodynamic, attachment, trauma, narrative and systemic ideas. The books are written in an accessible and readable style with a focus on practice. Each text offers theoretical background and guidance for practice, with creative use of clinical examples.

Arlene Vetere, Professor of Family Therapy and Systemic Practice at VID Specialized University, Oslo, Norway.

Rudi Dallos, Emeritus Professor, Dept. of Clinical Psychology, University of Plymouth, UK.

Siv Merete Myra · Tone Grøver · Ulf Axberg
Editors

New Horizons in Systemic Practice with Children and Families

palgrave
macmillan

Editors
Siv Merete Myra
Department of Family Therapy
and Systemic Practice
Faculty of Social Studies
VID Specialized University
Oslo, Norway

Tone Grøver
Department of Family Therapy
and Systemic Practice
Faculty of Social Studies
VID Specialized University
Oslo, Norway

Ulf Axberg
Department of Family Therapy
and Systemic Practice
Faculty of Social Studies
VID Specialized University
Oslo, Norway

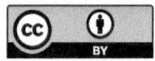

ISSN 2662-9127   ISSN 2662-9135   (electronic)
Palgrave Texts in Counselling and Psychotherapy
ISBN 978-3-031-38110-2   ISBN 978-3-031-38111-9   (eBook)
https://doi.org/10.1007/978-3-031-38111-9

Cover illustration: © Sergey Ryumin/Getty Images

This Palgrave Macmillan imprint is published by the registered company Springer Nature Switzerland AG
The registered company address is: Gewerbestrasse 11, 6330 Cham, Switzerland

Acknowledgements

Behind a book there is always a great we. This book is no exception. Thanks to a wide range of contributors, we were able to start and finish this work. First and foremost, we want to give our deepest thanks to Jim Sheehan and Arlene Vetere. For years they have been an enormous inspiration and have made many contributions to our systemic family therapist milieu at VID Specialized University. They have also helped us connect with other systemic milieus as well as publishers in Europe. Quite simply, this book wouldn't have come into existence at all if it wasn't for them and their overwhelming generosity in their guiding of us.

We want also to express our gratitude to all our collaboration partners who seek to relate to their own lives, together with us, in what we call therapy rooms. Their living presence shows up, anonymized, in different parts of the chapters in this book. From them we have learned more than is possible to learn from any book. Without the inspiration received from them, this book would be empty in both a real and metaphorical sense. As readers will see, rich contributions were received from all who supported this work by allowing themselves to be interviewed and by sharing their own time and insights with the authors.

We also want to thank VID Specialized University in Oslo, especially our Head of Studies Halvor de Flon and Dean Mona-Iren Hauge, for giving the space, support and time needed to complete this work. The editors also owe a great debt to our professional 'godfathers', Per Jensen and Håkon Hårtveit, who established our systemic family therapy education in Oslo. Thanks to their pioneering work, it has grown from a few enthusiastic people walking around in slippers to one of Europe's largest systemic training programmes.

Last but not least our gratitude goes to our friends, families, partners and pets! They are there, for inspiration and insight, reminding us, every day, about how dependent we are on each other, giving inspiration to go deeper into the complexity and beauty of systemic understanding.

One final acknowledgement of dependence: all that is written here in this book by editors and authors rests on the shoulders of our wonderful colleagues, past and present, both from systemic milieus and from other disciplines. In systemic spirit, we don't want to make division between disciplines, and this richness is one of the reasons why we are so grateful to be part of systemic understanding.

With love,

Siv Merete Myra
Tone Grøver
Ulf Axberg

Contents

Notes on Contributors

Ulf Axberg Ph.D. is a professor in Family Therapy and Systemic Practice at the VID Specialized University in Oslo, Norway. In addition, he is a licensed psychologist and psychotherapist and clinical supervisor. He has long experience working in Child and Adolescent Mental Health and Social Services. His main research interests are systemic intervention, parental support and children exposed to intimate partner violence. He has authored and co-authored several articles in peer-reviewed journals and book chapters.

Esben Esther Pirelli Benestad (EEPB) is Cand. Med. Family therapist IAP, specialist in clinical sexology NACS and professor emeritus in sexology at the University of Agder, Norway. EEPB has since 1985 worked both as a researcher and as clinician for the transgender and gender diverse (TGD) population in addition to working as a GP for more than 40 years. Being a transgifted individual themselves, EEPB has had the unique option to see the TGD population and all their networks through several perspectives.

Halvor de Flon is associate professor and programme coordinator at VID Specialized University, Oslo, is a nurse and has a master's degree in systemic family therapy. He has worked about 30 years with families and couples within child and adolescent psychiatry as family therapist and leader of family services. He has participating in innovation and development of different family-based services. He has published scientific book—chapters about supervision, family therapy, education of family therapists and reflecting team and processes.

Anne Grasaasen is associate professor at VID Specialized University, Oslo where she teaches family therapy to masters' level students. In addition to teaching and supervising, she is also currently affiliated with Samtalesenteret, a free therapy practice, run by the students. Her main research interests are about family as phenomenon and family life. She also concerned about research into pedagogy related to education, and how to make students ready work as a family therapist with a sense of mastery and relevant knowledge. She also has extensive clinical practice as a family therapist on medical paediatric wards for many years, with families and children in the addiction field.

Tone Grøver is an associate professor at VID Specialized University, Oslo, is a sociologist, has a master's degree in systemic family therapy and has a specialist education in narrative psychotherapy. She has worked for over 20 years as a private therapist for couples, families and individuals. She has also worked on assignments for the public and private sector with conflicts, work environment challenges and conversations with managers (coaching) for almost 30 years. She has published three works of fiction, and in her teaching, she emphasizes a narrative form. She is interested in the insights we gain in therapy through art and poetic language.

Gina Hægland is clinical psychologist and family therapist. She has been working with children, youth and their families in different parts of the health services since 2001. She has been teaching family therapy for 11 years and has a lot of experience with systemic supervision in different constellations. She has been professionally responsible for an education programme in family therapy for six years. Today she is working as an clinical psychologist in an outpatient unit with eating disorders.

Siv Merete Myra is associate professor at VID Specialized University, Oslo, Norway, since 2014. She completed her postgraduate dissertation in 2018 with the University of Oslo, Faculty of Medicine. She is a member of the Faculty of Social Studies at VID Specialized University where she teaches family therapy to masters' level students. She has been working in specialized health care for 25 years with families and children in the addiction field. She supervises therapists in the field of addiction, child welfare and family therapy. Her primary systemic practice interest is children and families living with substance abuse disorder and the prevention of intergenerational transference. Her research has been related to pregnant substance-abusing women in compulsory and voluntary treatment settings in Norway, and their therapists.

Bill Petitt has a master's degree in social work and is a licensed psychotherapist and clinical supervisor in psychotherapy. He has his own training institute and for more than forty years he has been active in training and supervising professionals working within social work, both adult and child psychiatry and education. His special interest is in the theoretical foundations of psychotherapy and in the philosophy of psychotherapy. He has written and co-authored many books and articles.

Marc van Roosmalen, Dr. is a Consultant Clinical Psychologist who works in child mental health services in Luton and South Bedfordshire East London Foundation Trust National Health Services, UK. His clinical and research interests are conceptualizing and operationalizing community-based services that are co-produced with communities, following a relational (or, systemic) and resilience approach to well-being. He uses theory of change and programme logic modelling to structure, deliver and evaluate the often complex community interventions.

Jim Sheehan is professor emeritus in family therapy and systemic practice at VID Specialized University, Oslo. He is a systemic family therapist, trainer and systemic supervisor with a background of more than 30 years of practice as a social worker. He lives and practises in the Republic of Ireland. His recent publications include *Family Conflict After Separation and Divorce* (2018, Palgrave) and two edited texts with Arlene

Vetere: *Long Term Systemic Therapy* (2020, Palgrave) and *Supervision of Family Therapy and Systemic Practice* (2017, Springer).

Vigdis Wie Torsteinsson is clinical psychologist, family therapist and philosopher. She has been working with children, youth and their families in different parts of the health services, from outreach services to family treatment centres and inpatient units. She has been teaching family therapy since 1995, the last years including Family-Based Therapy for eating disorders. She has been an editor of the Nordic family therapy journal (Fokus på familien) for two periods, and has written several books, articles and chapters on family therapy, developmental psychology and eating disorders.

List of Figures

1

Editors Introduction

Siv Merete Myra, Tone Grøver, and Ulf Axberg

This book will illustrate how systemic theory, as both a meta-theory and a relational organic theory, can be a suitable framework for understanding and appreciating the new horizons of systemic practice with children and families in their various contexts. Even if our ambition is to present new horizons in systemic therapy, we also gratefully acknowledge the influences from earlier systemic authors, therapists and researchers whose contributions are made visible in the various chapters. In acknowledging

S. M. Myra (✉) · U. Axberg
Department of Family Therapy and Systemic Practice, Faculty of Social
Studies, VID Specialized University, Oslo, Norway
e-mail: siv.merete.myra@vid.no

U. Axberg
e-mail: ulf.axberg@vid.no

T. Grøver
Department of Family Therapy and Systemic Practice, Faculty of Social
Studies, VID Specialized University, Oslo, Norway
e-mail: Tone.Grover@vid.no

© The Author(s) 2024
S. M. Myra et al. (eds.), *New Horizons in Systemic Practice with Children
and Families*, Palgrave Texts in Counselling and Psychotherapy,
https://doi.org/10.1007/978-3-031-38111-9_1

the importance of the contribution to the systemic field of many earlier authors, we hope to show how we need a place on which we can stand and watch in order to see the (new) horizons.

The chapters in the present book are written at a time of profound changes and many challenges, such as, climate changes, wars and pandemic, creating uncertainty but also many possibilities. In all this, the complex nature of dynamic systems becomes very visible. Systemic thinking encourages, maybe even requires a plurality of theories, perspectives and approaches. Indeed, as Axberg and Petitt write in one of their chapters, referencing Luigi Onnis, the keyword in the paradigm of complexity is plurality. But also, a systemic perspective is a way of understanding our being in the world, from the big questions to the small choices we make together. For example, Myra illustrates in her chapter how even small therapeutic interventions can be of vital importance in complex situations.

The different chapters shed light on how systemic perspectives, as they are presented in their varying contexts, hopefully promote hope by giving room for reflections on uncertainty, change, opportunities, interconnections and differences. Furthermore, the chapters will foreshadow the ways that systemic theory makes space for a multiplicity of varying approaches that addresses the needs of children and those assisting them in their different settings, where children grow and develop in the context of their unique needs and challenges. Importantly we can see this systemic influence even in settings where other perspectives are prevailing.

So why do we need this book about new horizons for systemic practice with children and families? Because we wanted to explore newer applications of our understanding of the developments in systemic practice and to show how a growing integration of research with these new developments across the broader fields of psychotherapy and counselling can be held within a systemic relational umbrella. In this book, we focus on the lives of children and families, organizations and staff that work with children. For example, working systemically with children and families in a medical context, with diagnostic practices and the dilemmas of labelling children, systemic consultation practices in social, health and educational contexts, the impact of separation and divorce on child and family development, working with parents in inpatient treatment displaying substance use problems, working systemically with disability, working with manualized approaches to eating disorders and with the intergenerational impacts of service responses. The emphasis in this book will be on the social utility of these new approaches, their historical origins, and how practice can be enhanced as a result. All the editors and authors are leading some of the developments in their particular field of competence. Several of the authors are affiliated with VID Specialized University, Oslo, which provides one of the largest systemic training programs in Europe. All the authors are using examples from systemic practice across a range of health and social care contexts.

In the first chapter, *Jim Sheehan* addresses the challenges for systemic approaches attempting to assist children and young people to navigate the often conflict-filled terrain of their parents' separation and divorce. He suggests that systemic interventions need to be fortified by a human rights perspective as practitioners aim to facilitate the continuation of childhood in the face of several forms of its interruption.

Next, Anne *Grasaasen and Esben Esther Benestad Pirelli* shed light over the understanding of gender as a phenomenon that is in major change. They reflect on how to create systemic conversations where children and youth, together with their families, in a safe context, can explore feelings and experiences about their gender identity.

In the following chapter, *Siv Merete Myra* addresses what kind of focus can be *large* enough in sessions with parents who have substance use problems. She shows how small interventions in complex situations can co-create a space that allows for the sharing of perspectives that can enable the parents to find a way forward together.

Anne Grasaasen describes in her chapter, meetings with families of children who have serious illnesses and where death has become the frame of family life. In encounters with parents dealing with anticipatory grief, therapists must also attempt to create alliances with scientific discourses. She illustrates the utility of systemic perspectives in a medical context by expanding causal explanations and providing descriptions of illness within a frame of relational values.

Thereafter, *Vigdis Wie Torsteinsson* and *Gina Hægland* wish to create some ideas about a new horizon in working within the framework of a manual. The Family-Based Treatment manual works as their example, but the points they underscore can be useful in any manualized context. They suggest a possible way to modify the manual without removing the efficient factors that have been the core of the positive results, by working with systemic formulation.

The chapters by Myra, Grasaasen, Torsteinsson and Hægland all describe the work in contexts where medical or psychiatric diagnoses are prominently in focus. *Ulf Axberg and Bill Petitt* address the question of whether systemic perspectives and psychiatric diagnoses are mutually exclusive or inclusive. Central to their systemic perspective is that systemic therapists also have a fundamental need to organize the domain of human suffering. It can bring order to clinical practice, research and professional communication, but crucially it will be in a parallel but different manner to the way in which it is important for medical practitioners.

The chapter from de Flon and Sheehan focuses on systemic work with families with children that have different and various kinds of difficulties that they have had since birth as a result of accidents and injuries. Illustrating systemic practice when the commonly underlaying assumption and expectation that problems in families and family living can and should be solved and forced to disappear is challenged.

The last two chapters of the book shed light on how systemic perspectives can be useful within the school context. In the chapter by *Marc van Roosmalen,* the Community Relations model (CoRe) is presented. It reconceptualizes a child mental health service, and how it can be operationalized. The CoRe model shifts from an individualized overwhelmingly deficit or illness model of mental health to a relational, resilience-based and integrated systems model that works systemically with partners and communities, with a focus on thriving communities and professional systems. Finally, in the chapter by *Ulf Axberg and Bill Petitt* the authors illustrate the idea that within a systemic framework it can be possible to encompass any idea that helps increase our understanding and effectiveness, even when it includes the combination of two separate intervention models, derived from very different philosophical and theoretical traditions.

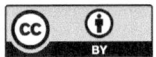

2

Systemic Approaches to Safeguarding Children's Rights Through Parental Separation and Divorce: Opening Spaces for Childhood to Continue

Jim Sheehan

Introduction

The concept of childhood informs most, if not all, chapters in this volume. While systemic practitioners take the concept for granted most of the time, a historical perspective allows us see that childhood, as understood in contemporary Western societies, has been an evolving concept that has seen many transitions in meaning over recent centuries (Aries, 1962; de Mause, 1974; Erikson, 1963). The idea of childhood functions today not simply as a descriptive concept laying out the features of the first significant segment of the human lifespan but as a concept imbued with a range of moral/practical imperatives addressed to all who interact and engage with those who enjoy the status of 'child'. For almost all Western states, this descriptive/moral journey reached a

J. Sheehan (✉)
Department of Family Therapy and Systemic Practice, Faculty of Social Studies, VID Specialized University, Oslo, Norway
e-mail: jimssheehan@outlook.com

© The Author(s) 2024
S. M. Myra et al. (eds.), *New Horizons in Systemic Practice with Children and Families*, Palgrave Texts in Counselling and Psychotherapy,
https://doi.org/10.1007/978-3-031-38111-9_2

point of culmination in the United Nations Convention on the Rights of the Child (1989). This convention defines the child as a person under the age of 18 years and declares the members of this group as subjects who are the bearers of many different rights which must be acknowledged and honoured by the states who are signatories to the Convention. The Convention acknowledges the family as the fundamental unit of society and puts emphasis on the role of parents as primary caregivers with responsibility for the upbringing of their children at the same time as obliging governments to support parents in fulfilling their essential role.

This chapter is about some of the different ways that systemic practitioners can and should play a part in the promotion and protection of children's wellbeing as they go through one of the most challenging transitions in family life, namely the separation and divorce of their parents. An explicit assumption of the chapter is that the work of systemic practitioners in this arena of family transition must be oriented not only towards the amelioration of children's psychological and relational suffering but, more importantly, towards the protection and promotion of the human rights that are theirs by virtue of belonging to the category of child. The current COVID-19 pandemic, which has seen many temporary changes and suspensions in the organization of children's lives, brings into focus many of those rights that have been taken for granted in many Western societies for a considerable period. These very suspensions of the 'normal' have provoked a deeper reflection on children's rights in all areas of their existence.

Three groups of rights highlighted in the Convention that have special relevance for the work considered in this chapter are children's *participation* rights, their rights to *provision* of those elements/resources necessary for their development and their *protection* rights. The first of these refers to their right to have an opinion and to have a say in matters affecting their own lives. The second concerns their right to education, play, leisure and cultural activities in addition to their right to access information. The third refers to their safeguarding and protection from all forms of abuse, neglect and exploitation. The chapter will progress in the following three sections which describe how different kinds of the separation/divorce transition, embodying different levels of conflict in the postseparation parenting relationship, can threaten children's rights in one way or another. The first section describes how the child's participation rights can be threatened even at the least conflictual end of the separation/divorce spectrum. The second section describes how a gradually more conflictual separation process puts at risk children's connection to resources that promote their development, while the third section describes how the performance of certain postseparation/divorce conflict life cycles embody the phenomenon of parental alienation as a form of emotional child abuse which threatens children's protection rights. Each section will consider some ways the systemic practitioner can intervene to restore children's rights when they are threatened or removed by circumstances beyond their control. While the contexts described in the three sections involve different levels of anxiety, disruption and harm in children's lives, the principal aim of systemic interventions is always the same, namely the restoration and continuation of childhood.

Promoting Children's Participation Rights in Transition Decisions

The great majority of separating parents have the goal of bringing their children through the separation/divorce transition with as little impact as possible. Notwithstanding these good intentions many fail to achieve this goal to different degrees and seek the assistance of the systemic practitioner through different avenues. For some, the desire to protect their children by creating as much certainty about the future as possible blinds them from the realization that children need timely access to information, given in an age-appropriate manner, if they are to have the opportunity to process an impending major change in their developing lives or to have an opportunity to express an opinion and have a say in decision-making processes that deeply impacts them and their futures. The task of the systemic practitioner engaged by such parents, either privately or through a social/health services agency, is not simply to support parents emotionally in their personal and relational crises or to provide them with developmentally relevant information about children and adolescents going through a parental separation or to help them mediate disputes about the division of their future childcare responsibilities. While all of these family-focused systemic interventions may be necessary, the practitioner must also assist by orienting or re-orienting parents towards their children as persons who have rights and entitlements as subject humans independent from themselves. Parents may be unaware of the way the states to which they belong enshrine in legislation or statutory protocols the rights of their children to information and participation. Or the states to which those parents belong may vary in the extent to which they foster awareness in parents and professionals of the rights of children under the UN Convention despite being signatories to the Convention.

Depending upon the degree of conflict between parents surrounding the separation decision, the systemic practitioner will also have a key role in assisting the parents, where possible, reach an agreement about an acceptable narrative to share with their children concerning the impending separation event and the reasons it is coming about. Intensive engagement with the systemic practitioner at this early stage in the separation process, where parents successfully mediate the narrative to be shared with their children and the means and timing of sharing it, can be enormously protective of children's current and future rights. It also augurs well for a less disrupted experience for children as well as for a shortening of the time in which their parents may remain in conflict and matters about the future remain uncertain. It is ironic, therefore, that the parents who most want to protect their children from the effects of their own conflict and use this desire as a momentum towards reaching an agreement about the future are often the parents who overlook their children's entitlement to have a say in the decision-making process. Hence, while being in receipt of the key piece of information that a separation is going to occur in addition to hearing a parentally agreed narrative concerning the separation decision goes some way to protecting children's rights to information in the context, it does not meet their right to participate in the decision-making process that accompanies such a major change in their life context. But how can and should systemic practitioners promote these child participation rights?

Child Participation in Decision-Making: The Positioning of Parents and Children

Family therapy, family mediation and child or adolescent therapies are often the contexts in which systemic practitioners encounter the separating family. These are the contexts, then, in which the practitioner must work out with family members what meaningful participation in decision-making might look like for each child. This is normally worked out initially with parents themselves and Sheehan (2018) has noted five basic positions that separating parents can adopt regarding the participation of their children in transition-related decision-making processes. Both parents may want child participation; neither parent may want such participation; one may want it and the other doesn't; both parents may want some children involved but not others; or both parents may be open to child participation but not until they have agreed the basic outlines of future custody and care arrangements. These positions are to be understood as starting parental positions which can and often do alter as dialogue with the practitioner evolves.

Where parents agree to child participation in the context of family mediation one of the first concerns of the systemic practitioner must be for the emotional safety of the child/adolescent throughout the process of their possible participation. This normally means having a consultation with the child/adolescent about their possible participation and the rules of engagement through which they might participate. This is not a simple matter and there can be many pitfalls accompanying a process that looks benign and child-focused on the surface. Children may already be triangulated into their parents' conflict in particular ways and may have different sets of fears and anxieties concerning their participation. They may already be in the middle of a grief process concerning the loss of family and may fear that the expression of their views and wishes could damage their relationship with one or both parents. Or they may fear being punished by one parent for the expression of certain views and wishes.

Eight different child/adolescent positions have been noted regarding their participation in the decision-making processes consequent upon the separation decision of their parents (Sheehan, 2018). As with their parents, these child positions may change across time and a critical skill required of the systemic practitioner engaged in the family mediation process is the ongoing negotiation between children and parents as their respective positions evolve. Child positions on participation include the following: the child who wants and expects participation from the outset and expects their voice to be the basis of their future reality; a child who is reluctant to participate because they fear rejection or punishment by one parent if their views and wishes were to become known; the child who wants to participate but only on the basis of their views never becoming known to their parents; the child who wants to be involved so that they can be as fully informed as possible about their parents' future plans without wishing to express any views themselves about their future; the child who wants to be as fully involved as possible with the intention of doing all they can to stop the separation process; the adolescent who wants limited participation in the decision-making process but simply wishes their parents to take note of their priorities—for example, the adolescent wants to use participation to say to her parents 'I don't mind how you work this out and I will go along with whatever you decide so long as I can still spend some time with my best friend every weekend'; a further position taken up by some children when offered opportunities to participate is a clear refusal to participate—it is as though the child says to both parents 'this is your decision to separate so you go and work out the details and don't burden me with having to be involved'; and, finally, a child may want to participate and may wish to express some views and perspectives so long as they can do so without their siblings or their parents becoming aware of their perspectives. While some children will refuse to meet with the family mediator others will use the child consultation to communicate their position with the practitioner and it is not uncommon that this position shifts within the context of a single consultation.

One of the most important rules of engagement attaching to children's possible participation is that surrounding the confidentiality they may require for their own emotional safety during an evolving family mediation process. Going slowly and carefully negotiating confidentiality arrangements between themselves and their parents is an important building block of a satisfactory process. The challenge for the systemic practitioner is to retain everyone's trust in the process as they move between and within a series of separate but connected dialogues involving different members of a separating family group. In particular, the practitioner needs to be clear about what child perspectives they have the child's permission to share with parents and what information and views the child does not want shared. A pitfall here can be that parents, at the outset of a process, can appear to completely agree that their child's views can be kept confidential in line with their child's wishes but then revert to a different position after their child has met with the practitioner and expressed some views. Practitioners can be met with a demand from parents to be told of their child's perspectives on the basis that 'we are her parents; we have a right to know'! It is important that practitioners do not break trust with child clients notwithstanding the pressure exerted upon them by anxious parents.

Child Participation: Communicating Reactions and Expressing Wishes

When thinking about child entitlements to participation in this context it can be helpful to think about two somewhat different aspects of this right to participation. The first aspect is the opportunity to *communicate their reactions* to someone who is competent to understand such reactions and to be supported in doing so while the second aspect concerns their opportunity to *express some wishes* about their future. This skill of providing an empathic and supportive response to the child's reactions to the new context they face is an important facet of the systemic practitioner's protection and promotion of child participation entitlements. Without it the child may never find within themselves the capacity to work out what they really want and to have a say in the decision-making processes impacting their future.

This distinction between providing receptive and empathic ears and eyes for children and the facilitating of their expression of wishes for their future is nowhere more relevant than when thinking of the participation entitlements of the very young child. Depending on their age and cognitive capacities, a young child may or may not be able to give voice to anything that resembles an expression of their wishes for the future. This does not mean, however, that they should be left out of therapeutic or mediation processes aimed at providing participation opportunities for their sibling group. The use of art and play therapy within family therapy and family mediation processes can provide the young child with the opportunity of communicating their reactions to a changed family environment (Gils, 2015) and can be one mechanism through which the systemic practitioner can honour the participation entitlements of the young child. The systemic practitioner does not have to be a qualified art or play therapist to engage creatively with the young child in the context of major family transition but they do need a commitment to making appropriate expressive spaces available to the young child and a conviction that the young child's participation entitlements are equal to those of their older siblings.

Reducing and Containing Postseparation Parental Conflict: Protecting the Developmental Rights of Children

When parents are unable to find their own agreement and require family court involvement to resolve their child-related disputes, this usually signals the breakdown of a number of different systems. It may signal a failure in one or both parents to *self-regulate* their own emotion and behaviour postseparation. In such contexts, uncontained anger and unresolved hurt and loss in one or both parents may move them along the path of their own desires alone to enact whatever they think is right themselves regardless of the position and wishes of their ex-partner/parent or the wishes of their children. This breakdown in the capacity to self-regulate in either one or both parents is inevitably accompanied by the breakdown of their capacity to *co-regulate* in the parental management and care of their children. This co-regulation may have operated effectively at previous points in their parenting and systemic interventions must always be aimed at the restoration of this capacity in time. However, when parental conflict and dispute reaches a certain level *external regulation* is usually required for a period to enable the re-establishment of the self-regulatory and co-regulatory capacities of family members and their relationships. This re-establishment can be assisted by a mixture of different external regulatory mechanisms which can include court orders relating to parent-child contact, engagement in parent education programmes aimed at the needs of separating parents, family therapy, individual therapies for parents and/or their children, and the appointment by the court of a parent coordinator who will have devolved upon them by the court certain decision-making functions in addition to mediating functions. All such external mechanisms are designed to protect children from the effects of certain levels of parental hostility, conflict and dispute which threaten their capacity to participate in the ordinary social institutions which foster their development in different ways. In the many different ways described in the paragraphs below children's developmental pathways are regularly interrupted and their capacities diminished in significant ways. Ongoing and poorly contained conflict between parents is usually the factor which impacts the child's capacity to benefit from the normal developmental opportunities available to them throughout different parts of their childhood (Lansford, 2009; Sheehan, 2020). A small selection of these conflicts affecting children at different stages in their development are described in the paragraphs below along with the systemic interventions that may allow for some protection of their developmental rights.

Parental Conflict and the Young Child: Systemic Responses

Parental conflict over the management of even *the very young child* can be enough to produce anxiety and uncertainty in the child as well as a very disrupted physical/bodily experience. It is not uncommon for the routine of the very young child to be the battleground on which separating parents play out their mutual hostilities. A refusal by parents to coordinate sleep and dietary patterns or to agree child safety strategies may ensure that the child suffers a very dysregulated experience which can show itself in problematic behaviour patterns in creche or school. Such behaviour patterns are likely to impact not only their own capacity to benefit from early learning experiences but also the opportunities available to their peers. From the child's point of view, at a very basic level, the lack of predictability surrounding their basic physical rhythms and requirements challenges their development of trust in the world around them, a factor which impacts all future development. While such parental failures may or may not attract the attention and strong intervention of child protection authorities, the systemic practitioner engaged to assist such parents and children may need to perform several functions. The may fulfil a very important educative role with parents concerning the impact on their child of their own dysregulated parental pattern; they may assist the parents in negotiating/mediating a resolution to their immediate parenting differences thereby removing the child and their development from the site on which their continuing interpersonal struggles are performed; they may be a source of referral for the parents for either individual therapy or may offer ongoing support to the conflictual parenting dyad to help them implement the terms of any agreed resolution. An essential part to the systemic assistance might also include some coaching for both parents with respect to developing respectful ways to communicate efficiently and effectively with each other regarding their ordinary day-to-day observations of, and concern for, their child. An example of such intervention might be the setting up of a diary system in which both parents might make entries and which would travel with the child between homes.

Parental Conflict and the Child Attending Elementary School: Systemic Responses

A very typical way in which the developmental rights of *the child attending elementary school (typically a child between the ages of 5 years and 12 years)* are threatened concerns the refusal by one parent to honour the social and sporting/recreational commitments that are already evolving in the child's life. A non-residential parent may feel they have too little quality time with their child and consequently be unwilling to share this time with the child's friends or with the child's activities. That parent may feel that such activities were organized for the child without reference to them and their needs and simply be unwilling to 'release' the child for participation in such activities during 'their' time. Children caught in such circumstances may even say to one parent that they miss engaging regularly in these activities while saying to another parent that it is not important to them whether they do or not. Whether the sacrifices such children make are imposed upon them or appear voluntarily made, the consequences are the same: they must forgo the opportunity to develop the strong bonds with their peers that are an outgrowth of a regular, shared participation as well as well as forgoing opportunities to learn and become proficient in the skill sets that are the focus of their surrendered activities. If such a pattern is not arrested at an early stage it can be the basis of a developing isolation within the adolescent's life and add a greater loading to the task of developing an appropriate level of autonomy and independence from both parents. The systemic practitioner informed by a children's rights focus will educate parents regarding what is at stake for the child in resolving certain dilemmas in particular ways. While organizing individual therapeutic support for the child if they are open to this, they may also attempt to convene the parents for a shared reflection on the child's position and a consideration of less costly ways of resolving the parental dilemmas and conflicts regarding parenting time. More specific court orders may be required for some parents and the systemic practitioner advising the court may have a critical role in the shaping of revised court orders.

A further very typical way that children's developmental rights are threatened in the postseparation phase of family life is through the experience of open hostility between their parents during 'handovers' of children from one parent to another. While it has been recognized for some time that exposure to high levels of interparental conflict has been more detrimental to children than parental divorce itself (Hetherington et al., 1998), studies have also identified that exposure to overt parental conflict (belligerence, contempt, derision, screaming, insulting, slapping, threatening and hitting) has been linked to externalizing problems in children while covert conflict (trying to get the child to side with one parent, using the child to get information about the other parent, using the child to carry messages to the other parent and denigrating the other parent in front of the child) has been more associated with the development of internalized problems (Buehler et al., 1998). Exposure to open parental conflict at the time of handovers will normally lead to anxiety, fear and apprehension in children for different lengths of time in advance of handovers and hand backs between their parents. The length of time children remain in the grip of these strong emotions can vary but without intervention the emotional impact of their exposure can be a significant detractor from their capacity to successfully engage both with their school curriculum and their out-of-school activities, both of which carry implications for their developmental rights. Where open parental conflict at handovers persists over time the anxiety for some children may reach such a level that they are simply not able to go on visits with their non-resident parent and will either be sick or say they do not wish to go without giving a specific reason for their position. While these latter situations can often be incorrectly understood as parental alienation (which will be described in more detail in the next section), they are primarily anxiety responses fuelled by persistent exposure to overt parental conflict.

What can the systemic practitioner do to protect the developmental rights of children in such situations? They can try to acknowledge and contain the parents' anger and hurt emotions (this may sometimes involve encouraging them to accept a therapeutic referral), offer them psychoeducational opportunities concerning the impact of their open conflict on their children, invite them to separate the event of handovers from the negotiation of all other parental business, and in the event of being unable to cease their open conflict in front of the children, to encourage them to structure the handovers in a way that does not involve them meeting each other (e.g. the collection of children from school, childminders or out-of-school activities). Where this cannot be negotiated successfully the systemic practitioner may play a part in advising the family court about the handover arrangements that are necessary for the protection of children. The systemic practitioner will also need to consider with parents the therapeutic needs of their children. This may be particularly relevant for the child whose heightened anxiety has led to a breakdown in the rhythm of their contact with the non-residential parent. The earliest interventions possible usually lead to the best outcomes for children.

Parental Conflict and the Adolescent: Systemic Responses

The developmental rights of *the adolescent* young person may be severely compromised by the ongoing conflict of their parents postseparation. The costs for adolescents may be experienced at the level of their developing autonomy, in the context of their school participation and achievement, or in the context of highly dysregulated emotional and behavioural patterns. Where parental conflict has been intense in the past and there have been hard-fought battles over care schedules for young children, adolescents may be the victims of their parents' incapacity to renegotiate care arrangements in the light of the young person's advancing years. It is not uncommon for 14- and 15-year-olds to be still adhering to care schedules that were made when they were 7 or 8 years old. The parental failure to open the care schedule to further consideration with the adolescent means that they continue to be caught in a conflict of loyalties and remain trapped in the fear that if they were to express some wishes that might be more in keeping with their evolving developmental needs they might ignite once more the currently dormant conflict between their parents as well as running the risk of being considered disloyal to one parent or the other. If unaddressed, such impasses can lead to the sacrificing of the kind of autonomy the young person needs for their social and personal development and such sacrifice may find its indirect expression in symptoms like self-harm gestures and/or suicidality. Or the adolescent may simply wish to spend some more time in the company and care of one parent and worry that the expression of such a desire will be misinterpreted by their other parent who may reject them.

A further conundrum arises for the adolescent caught in a cross generational coalition (Haley, 1973) with their residential parent against their non-residential parent. In this type of family configuration, the young person is covertly asked to side with one parent against the other parent. The setting of rules and boundaries for the developing young person often becomes the battle ground between the parents with the young person being covertly rewarded for ignoring the appropriate limits set by the other parent on their behaviour. If unaddressed, this type of coalition formation can lead to poor school performance and/or attendance in the young person who may become more vulnerable to substance abuse and other risk behaviours as they become more disconnected from school and other structured out-of-school activities. In such contexts, the young person's developmental rights are sacrificed and the parent engaging in the covert invitation of the young person into alliance against the other parent may have little or no insight into their own behaviour.

A major contribution from the systemic practitioner in the context of many adolescent reactions to postseparation parental conflict is psychoeducation with the young person's parents. Parents may be unaware that their young person is caught in a conflict of loyalties and may be unaware that their own conflict-based rigidities are undermining their young person's developmental needs for more autonomy and more intense social engagement. They often need to be assisted to distinguish normal gender-based affinities that are emerging for the adolescent from the alienating behaviours that can be part of a coalition process that pulls a young person away from one parent. Where possible, the therapeutic convening of parents around the young person's needs for support, containment and supervision may go some way towards arresting familial and adolescent processes that are going out of control. The adolescent should always be encouraged, but not coerced, to avail of some extrafamilial support for themselves as well as encouraged, but not coerced, to engage therapeutically with both their parents either together or separately. Their risk behaviours, if these have developed, along with changing family dynamics need to be a focus of all the different systemic therapeutic engagements.

Parental Alienation and Children's Protection Rights: New Horizons for Systemic Practice

The title of this two-volume series points to newly emerging horizons within systemic practice. Within the practice domain under consideration in this chapter, new horizons are nowhere more evident than in that space where the most intense and prolonged postseparation parental disputes about children occur. These disputes usually involve some version of what specialists call the 'resist/refuse dynamic'(Walters & Friedlander, 2016)). This dynamic is seen in a group of children who show reluctance to go on court-ordered access/contact with their non-resident parent, resist meaningful engagement with this parent when they do go on court-prescribed visitation and sometimes refuse to have any contact whatsoever with that parent. For many years family courts and systemic practitioners have tried to address these issues through a mixture of parent education, child therapies and family therapy. Sometimes this mixture of interventions proved helpful with the relatively mild forms of this dynamic but failed spectacularly with the moderate to severe end of the postseparation conflict continuum. While the resist/refuse dynamic was descriptive of behavioural patterns displayed by a child, the family relational context in which the most severe expressions of the dynamic was usually embedded was better captured by the term 'parental alienation'. While the phenomenon has been recognized by child and family professionals for the last eighty years, it was not until the mid-1980's that Gardner (1985) coined the term *parental alienation syndrome*. Following a debate between clinicians over whether terminology should just be descriptive of a child's position/condition or whether it should reach towards more relational meanings, the field has now settled for the term *parental alienation* (Lorandos et al., 2013) which captures both individual and family relational dimensions.

Parental alienation should be understood as a type of *diagnosis* in the sense that Axberg and Pettit (see Chapter 9, this volume), drawing on earlier Greek meanings, give to that term, namely 'learning the phenomenon well, so that we can decide what kind it is'. For the DSM-5 of the American Psychiatric Association, the diagnostic label of 'Parent–Child Relational Problem' can be used whenever a child has been exposed to parental alienation strategies that are likely to cause 'unwarranted feelings of estrangement' in the child towards the targeted parent (American Psychiatric Association, 2013, p. 715). The alternative diagnostic label of 'Child Affected by Parental Relationship Distress' is offered by the ICD-10 when 'the negative effects of parental relationship discord (e.g., high levels of conflict, distress, or disparagement') are having a negative impact on the child. In the interests of 'learning the phenomenon well', this section of the chapter will now outline in more detail what parental alienation is and is not and will describe how it functions simultaneously as a unique and complex form of emotional child abuse and family violence. As a form of emotional child abuse, parental alienation brings the issue of children's protection rights under the UN Convention sharply into focus. The failure to address the issue in the context of parental disputes within family court systems undermines these rights and places children at risk for a range of negative short-term and long-term consequences. The positive and hopeful news is that when adequately addressed in a timely manner the systemic practitioner can play a decisive role in honouring the protection rights of children in the face of the phenomenon.

Parental Alienation and Parental Estrangement

Parental alienation can be described as a psychological condition in which a child strongly allies themselves with an alienating parent, often referred to as the 'preferred 'parent, and rejects a relationship with the alienated parent, often referred to as the 'targeted' parent, without legitimate justification (Harman et al., 2019). It often arises in family contexts where a more powerful parent engages in abusive behaviours designed to damage and destroy the relationship between the other less powerful parent and the child (Harman et al., 2018). As a relational scenario it must be distinguished from the kind of high conflict situations described in the previous section where both parents contribute relatively equally to creating a conflictual environment which can be very damaging to children in the different ways we have seen. Unlike the child victims of those conflict scenarios who suffer loyalty conflict, the child victims of parental alienation exhibit a range of behaviours first identified by Gardner (1992). They engage in a campaign of denigration against the non-resident parent; they offer weak, frivolous or absurd rationalizations for their denigrations; they portray a marked lack of ambivalence wherein all things to do with the denigrated parent are judged bad and all aspects of their favoured parent are judged good; the child claims their views about the targeted parent are theirs alone and are in no way influenced by their favoured parent; they display an absence of guilt for their actions and attitudes towards the targeted parent; they employ borrowed scenarios about past events to justify their positions, often recalling events that occurred before they were born as though they were direct eye witnesses; and they often extend their campaign of denigration against the targeted parent to include the targeted parent's extended family and friends.

If the above captures the essence of what parental alienation is when considered from the perspective of the child's presentation, this must be carefully distinguished by the systemic practitioner from what it is not. Parental alienation does not encompass situations where a child rejects a parent and refuses contact with them because of problems associated with that parent–child relationship itself. For example, if a child has experienced abusive behaviours from a parent or has been the recipient of neglect or poor parenting practices by that parent, the child's rejection of that parent can be described as *parental estrangement* or justified rejection. While the primary causes of parental alienation are the set of alienating behaviours (words and actions) performed by the alienating parent with a view to influencing the child to foreclose their relationship with the targeted parent, the central cause of parental estrangement is the past behaviour, whether neglectful or abusive or inadequate, of the now rejected parent.

Alienating Behaviours and Parental Alienation

While a very large number of alienating behaviours (e.g. badmouthing the other parent in front of the child, engaging in coercive controlling behaviours to force an alliance with the child and to reject the targeted parent, telling the child that the other parent does not love them, telling the child the other parent wishes to take them away for good from them, confiding in the child about adult matters such as family finance or past sexual matters, limiting the child's contact with the other parent, consistently breaching court orders regarding contact time and communication with the other parent, giving the child 'permission' to choose to go on court-ordered contact periods or not and making false allegations of child abuse) have been documented by many researchers over the last two decades (Baker & Darnall, 2006; Harman et al., 2018) the identification of parental alienation as a complex form of family violence has happened more recently (Clawar & Rivlin, 2013; Harman et al., 2018; Haines et al., 2020). For these later researchers, parental alienation results from an alienating parent's coercion, control and generation of fear in a child towards the targeted parent. The performance of these behaviours constitutes a form of emotional abuse for child victims of parental alienation and a form of intimate partner violence inflicted by the alienating parent upon the targeted parent. Taken together, both realities make parental alienation a complex but significant child protection matter and an arena where children's rights under the UN Convention to protection from all forms of abuse are seriously compromised.

Impact of Parental Alienation

While more is known about the impact of parental alienation on targeted parents (they are an easier group for researchers to access than alienated children) than on their children, there is a growing body of evidence in both areas. Parent victims of parental alienation appear to suffer similar impacts to victims of other forms of intimate partner violence. These parents report experiencing depression (Taylor-Potter, 2015), anxiety and high levels of suicidality (Baker & Verrochio, 2015; Balmer et al., 2018) in addition to their ongoing experience of living with unresolved grief and ambiguous loss (Boss, 2016). Alienated children have been shown to suffer from more psychosocial adjustment disorders than children who have not been alienated and the effects of alienating behaviours associated with lengthy separations from the targeted parent have been associated with poor psychological adjustment in this group. Some research examining the longer-term impacts on adults who have been the victims of parental alienation as children (Baker, 2005; Ben-Ami & Baker, 2012; Baker & Verrocio, 2013) have shown that this group has experienced low levels of self-esteem and high levels of self-hatred, insecure attachment, substance abuse disorders, guilt, anxiety and depression. A more recent qualitative study (Bentley & Matthewson, 2020) of adult children's experience of parental alienation gives increased support to the above findings. Their participants reported experiencing anxiety, depression, low self-worth, guilt, attachment problems and difficulty in other relationships, in addition to delayed career or educational attainment. Some of the participants in the same study spoke of missing out on a childhood and their experience of an early loss of innocence. Clinicians treating adults who were sexually abused as children will be aware of the similarity in such experiences between the two groups.

So, what can this ever-expanding picture of parental alienation mean for systemic practitioners and, more particularly, for systemic intervention? The systemic practitioner may be in the role of an assessor for, and advisor to, the family court. Or the systemic practitioner may be in the role of family therapist treating the family system following an order of the family court for such treatment/therapy. The requirements of each role are different. In the first assessment/advisory role, the task is to make a diagnosis of parental alienation when this is warranted and to advise the court about its consequences for the child and best practices for its management and possible reversal. In the second role, the systemic practitioner is in the role of family therapist providing a unique form of family therapy which will be described below in addition to making updating reports on the progress of the therapy for both the court and the systemic practitioner in the assessment/advisory role. We will look here at what is involved in both systemic practitioner roles.

Diagnosing Parental Alienation

The systemic assessor will need to consider whether a diagnosis of parental alienation is warranted in any particular context. While there have been a host of different studies in recent decades contributing to a strong evidence-base for parental alienation the most comprehensive model for the diagnosis of parental alienation has been provided by Bernet (2020). His model suggests that five different factors need to be present for such a diagnosis to be made. These five factors are as follows: that the child manifests an avoidance of relationship with one of their parents; that there is evidence of a prior positive relationship between the child and the now rejected parent; that there is an historic absence of abuse, neglect or seriously deficient parenting on the part of the now rejected parent; that there is evidence of the use of multiple alienating behaviours on the part of the favoured parent; and that the child exhibits many of the eight behavioural manifestations of alienation initially identified by Gardner (1985). When these factors are present the systemic practitioner needs to be clear in their identification of parental alienation for the court and inform the court of the evidence surrounding both its short-term and longer-term consequences for the child. The second thing they must do is to propose an intervention strategy oriented towards the restoration of the child's relationship with the targeted parent with the longer-term goal of ensuring that the child's right to a relationship with both parents is protected. Regarding the intervention strategy the practitioner must assess whether there is a reasonable chance of restoration happening without the removal of the child from the care of the alienating parent. Family courts are justifiably hesitant to remove children from what has been their primary residence with their primary carer without sufficient cause. However, the practitioner will need to explain to the court that parental alienation is one of the contexts where such removal may be required for the protection of the child from the emotional abuse that is currently being perpetrated on the child. Where the assessor judges that there is a reasonable chance that a restoration path can be pursued successfully without a change of residence, they will often recommend a package psychoeducational and family therapy interventions to be delivered within a clear timeframe. For such family therapy interventions to be meaningful, it is essential that minimum progress goals are identified by the court for the parents and that the court manages and responds to the progress/lack of progress of the therapy in a timely fashion. A sense of urgency needs to be maintained by the assessor and the court as is fitting in any context where a child is being abused or neglected in any way.

Parental Alienation and a Specialized Form of Family Therapy

What does family therapy look like in this context? As many researchers (Haines et al., 2019; Templer et al., 2017) and specialist clinicians (Smith, 2016) have observed, family therapy in the treatment of parental alienation usually does not mean conjoint work with parents and child. Rather, it means work with each part of the family separately but simultaneously and conducted by the same therapist with different goals attaching to each part of the work. This does not mean that conjoint work between the parents themselves or between both parents and the child may not be fruitful in time and at different times of the work and the family therapist will have to judge if and when the time for such joint work has arrived.

What are the goals of such specialized family therapy? While the specific goals will vary from case to case the general goals of the therapy for the favoured/aligned parent are as follows: to enhance their support for a renewed relationship between their child and the targeted parent; to increase their awareness of their own ongoing alienating behaviours and to encourage the complete cessation of such behaviours; fostering an enhanced understanding of the psychological position of their child; and encouraging a greater level of sharing of information about the child with the targeted parent. The general goals for the therapeutic meetings with the child are to increase the child's understanding of the situation they finds themselves in, to restore a level of ambivalence in their thinking about both parents by challenging their distorted thinking and strengthening their critical thinking, as well as supporting them as they take their first steps in a renewed relationship with the targeted parent. There may be multiple facets of the therapeutic work with the targeted/alienated parent. These facets may include some or all of the following: providing an empathic ear with respect to the hurt and anger they feel concerning a range of false allegations that may have been made against them; helping them to separate these understandable feelings from the emotional charge they will experience as they commence a reunification process with their child who they may not have seen for a very long time; helping them to understand the complexity of the emotional situation their child has been in and that the emotional range of their child is much broader than the thin spectrum of feelings represented in their child's rejecting and denigrating behaviours; helping them to reflect on appropriate parental responses to their children who are trying to adapt to a massive change in their circumstances and who can only have a very limited understanding how such change is in their interest; encouraging them to overcome some of the social isolation that often goes with the territory of being an alienated/targeted parent; and assisting them to realize that they must now work to communicate effectively with the child's other parent even though there has been a long history of that parent refusing/failing to communicate with them.

Where the court, on the advice of the systemic assessor, decides that the child should have a change of residence if they are to have an opportunity to restore their relationship with the targeted parent, such decision usually comes about as a result of the assessor's view that the alienating parent shows little or no insight into their alienating behaviour and shows little or no sign of willingness to assist in the restoration of the child's relationship with the targeted parent. In these contexts, the restoration path may only have an opportunity to be effective if the alienating parent is debarred from contact with the child for a couple of months or at least until such time as the child has re-established a positive relationship with the rejected parent. At that point, the court will have to decide, following advice from the assessor who has consulted with the family therapist, whether renewed contact between the child and the alienating parent should be supervised or unsupervised. Such decision will be wholly based upon the therapist's perception of that parent's willingness and capacity to desist from the alienating behaviours that have been a central part of the child's emotional abuse in the first place. Sometimes the change of residence in conjunction with the specialized form of family therapy described above leads over time to a place where the child's relationship with both parents is restored and sometimes it does not. The net outcome, however, even in these latter situations, is that the child has been protected from ongoing emotional abuse.

Conclusion

This chapter has adopted a children's rights perspective in the consideration of what systemic intervention can achieve in the face of post-separation parental conflict. It has described some typical ways in which children's participation, development and protection rights are compromised in the context of their parents' conflict during and following the separation/divorce process. It has also shown how different aspects of these rights may be compromised across the whole spectrum of postseparation family conflict, from the least conflictual separation to some of the most profound, lengthy and destructive postseparation family struggles. In keeping with the theme of the volume, the final section of the chapter has highlighted the new horizons emerging for the identification, management and treatment of the most severe forms of parental alienation which must be understood as a complex form of family violence, containing a combination of the emotional abuse of a child with a unique form of intimate partner violence. All familial processes described portray different kinds of disruption to childhood at different stages of child development and the stakes for systemic interventions have been seen to be the restoration and continuation of childhood.

References

American Psychiatric Association. (2013). *Diagnostic and statistical manual of mental disorders* (5th ed.). Author.

Aries, P. (1962). *Centuries of childhood: A social history of family life*. Trans. Robert Baldick.

Baker, A. J. L. (2005). The long-term effects of parental alienation on adult children: A qualitative research study. *The American Journal of Family Therapy, 33*, 289–302.

Baker, A. J. L. (2020). Reliability and validity of the four-factor model of parental alienation. *Journal of Family Therapy, 42*, 100–118.

Baker, A. J. L., & Darnall, D. (2006). Behaviours and strategies employed in parental alienation: A survey of parental experiences. *Journal of Divorce and Remarriage, 45*(1/2), 55–75.

Baker, A. J. L., & Verrocio, M. C. (2013). Italian college student-reported childhood exposure to parental alienation: Correlates with wellbeing. *Journal of Divorce and Remarriage, 54*, 609–628.

Baker, A. J. L., & Verrochio, M. C. (2015). Parental bonding and parental alienation as correlates of psychological maltreatment in adults in intact and non-intact families. *Journal of Child and Family Studies, 24*, 3047–3057.

Balmer, S., Matthewson, M., & Haines, J. (2018). Parental alienation: Targeted parent perspective. *Australian Journal of Psychology, 70*, 91–99.

Ben-Ami, N., & Baker, A. J. L. (2012). The long-term correlates of childhood exposure to parental alienation on adult self-sufficiency and wellbeing. *The American Journal of Family Therapy, 40*, 169–183.

Bentley, C., & Matthewson, M. (2020). The not-forgotten child: Alienated adult children's experience of parental alienation. *The American Journal of Family Therapy, 48*(5), 509–529.

Bernet, W. (2020, Summer). The five-factor model for the diagnosis of parental alienation. *Feedback: Journal of the Family Therapy Association of Ireland*, 3–15.

Boss, P. (2016). The context and process of theory development: The story of ambiguous loss. *Journal of Family Theory and Review, 8*, 269–286.

Buehler, C., Krishnakumar, A., Stone, G., Anthony, C., Pemberton, S., Gerard, J., & Barber, B.K. (1998). Interparental conflict styles and youth problem behaviors: A two-sample replication study. *Journal of Marriage and the Family, 60*, 119–132.

Clawar, S. S., & Rivlin, V. B. (2013). *Children held hostage: Identifying brainwashed children, presenting a case, and crafting solutions* (2nd ed.). American Bar Association.

de Mause, L. (Ed.). (1974). *The history of childhood*. Harper.

Erikson, E. H. (1963). *Childhood and Society* (2nd Ed.). Norton.

Gardner, R. (1985). Recent trends in divorce and custody litigation. *Academy Forum, 29*(2), 3–7.

Gardner, R. (1992). *The parental alienation syndrome: A guide for mental health and legal professionals*. Creative Therapeutics.

Gils, E. (2015). *Play in family therapy*. Guilford.

Haines, J., Matthewson, M., & Turnbull, M. (2019). *Understanding and managing parental alienation: A guide to assessment and intervention*. Routledge.

Haines, J., Matthewson, M., & Turnbull, M. (2020). *Understanding and Managing Parental Alienation: A Guide to Assessment and Intervention*. Routledge.

Haley, J. (1973). Toward a theory of pathological systems. In G. H. Zuk & I. Boszormenyi-Nagy (Eds.), *Family therapy and disturbed families* (pp. 11–27). Science and Behaviour Books.

Harman, J. J., Bernet, W., & Harman, J. (2019). Parental alienation: The blossoming of a field of study. *Current Directions in Psychological Science, 28*(2), 212–217.

Harman, J. J., Kruk, E., & Hines, D. A. (2018). Parental alienating behaviours: An unacknowledged form of family violence. *Psychological Bulletin, 144*(12), 1275–12999.

Hetherington, E.M., Bridges, M., & Insabella, G.M. (1998). What matters? What does not? Five perspectives on the association between marital transitions and children's adjustment. *American Psychologist, 53*, 167–184.

Lansford, J. E. (2009). Parental divorce and children's adjustment. *Perspectives on Psychological Science, 4*(2), 140–152.

Lorandos, D., Bernet, W., & Sauber, S. R. (Eds.). (2013). *Parental alienation: The handbook for mental health and legal professionals.* Charles C Thomas.

Sheehan, J. (2018). *Family conflict after separation and divorce: Mental health professional interventions in changing societies.* Palgrave.

Sheehan, J. (2020). The life cycles of family conflict after separation and divorce: A proposed typology. *Feedback: Journal of the Family Therapy Association of Ireland*, Summer, 43–63.

Smith, L. S. (2016). Family-based therapy for parent-child re-unification. *Journal of Clinical Psychology: in Session, 72*(5), 498–512.

Taylor-Potter, S. (2015.) *Effects of past parental alienation and ongoing estrangement from adult children on non-custodial parents as they age.* Available from ProQuest Dissertations and Theses Global.

Templer, K., Matthewson, M., Haines, J., & Cox, G. (2017). Recommendations for best practice in response to parental alienation: Findings from a systematic review. *Journal of Family Therapy, 39*, 103–122.

United Nations. (1989). *United Nations Convention on the Rights of the Child*.

Walters, M. G., & Friedlander, S. (2016). When a child rejects a parent: Working with the intractable resist/refuse dynamic. *Family Court Review, 54*(3), 424–445.

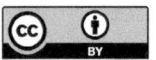

3

Gender Incongruence: Youth with a Special Talent for Gender; Supporting Youth and Families

Anne Grasaasen and Esben Esther Pirelli Benestad

Sarah: I feel like a boy. I've always felt this way. But now everything's all wrong.

Sarah is 13 years old. In the waiting room sit Mum and Dad. In the last conversation, we all participated, but this developed into a loud, somewhat aggressive exchange that was hard to land in a good way. Now Sarah does not want them to be included. She is dressed like most teenagers in jeans and a hoody, but I sense all the same that her low-hanging jeans and oversize sweater are not accidental choices.

Sarah: I've gotten breasts. I don't want them. I see them in the mirror every day and cry. I'm so tired of not feeling good. Every time

A. Grasaasen (✉)
Department of Family Therapy and Systemic Practice, Faculty of Social Studies, Oslo, Norway
e-mail: anne.grasaasen@vid.no

E. E. P. Benestad
University of Agder, Kristiansand, Norway

© The Author(s) 2024
S. M. Myra et al. (eds.), *New Horizons in Systemic Practice with Children and Families*, Palgrave Texts in Counselling and Psychotherapy,
https://doi.org/10.1007/978-3-031-38111-9_3

> someone shouts my name, I feel sick. I don't want to be called
> Sarah anymore, it's not me. I've been born in the wrong body.

As she struggles to find words, I sense that this is important to say. When
I ask how she wants things to be and how life could look then, she looks
at me with a serious gaze and whispers:

> Mum will never allow what I want. But I can't stand to wait until I'm
> 18.

Throughout the past decade, gender identity has had considerable
presence in the public debate. Questioning one's gender, identifying as
non-binary, agender or gender-fluid has become more usual. Though
not a new phenomenon, there is now broader social acknowledgement,
and this has produced challenges to our assumptions about nature and
culture (Butler et al., 2022). People experiencing a different gender identity than that assigned to them at birth are today standing up and
demanding their place in society. The contents of their demands range
from what the health service should provide to which changing room
they should be allowed to use. Over time, a space has opened in which
increasing numbers of people grappling with feelings of incongruence
between experienced gender identity and that assigned at birth have
helped to raise this issue. They tell stories of desires and needs, about
experiences of a narrow, gender-divided world in which they do not
feel at home. Various institutions, from the Crown to the Church,
from political leaders to schoolteachers have embraced the rainbow's
many colours to promote ideas of diversity, inclusion, the right to love
whomever one wants and to decide who one is. In many ways, this
has brought change and greater acceptance to areas of human life that
previously were tabu. New knowledge has also changed professional and
ethical thinking about children, youth and gender incongruence, and
many boundaries have been moved. The most common understanding
of the significant increase in youth choosing gender confirmative treatment is greater acceptance in many countries and those experiencing
gender incongruence to a greater extent finding the strength and courage
to promote their needs in fellowship (Coleman et al., 2022).

The view of trans identity as the desire to be "the opposite" gender has been challenged by increasing awareness of different non-binary identities (Butler, 2018). A quick internet search reveals many possible gender categories, and this list is expanding. While there has been an explosion in scientific research attempting to explain the increase in youths questioning their gender identities, there is less exploration of their lived experiences. It is the exception also in a therapeutic context to describe gender incongruence from the inside (Butler et al., 2022). Instead, these knowledge gaps are largely filled by information from social media and other internet platforms offering advice and guidance. The increasing openness about gender identity issues makes necessary an expansion of the conversational space with new ideas. The competence of the therapist regarding knowledge of gender attitudes and values is continuously on trial. We locate a pragmatic and culture-oriented perspective as the basis for understanding identities and concepts concerning gender. This involves the need to understand gender and gender understanding as phenomena that change over time, but that are stable enough in a cultural context to provide meaning and identity opportunities for people's lives and life worlds (Andersen & Malterud, 2013). We recognize identities as changeable and made possible by culture and society. We also acknowledge that categories can help people understand themselves and cope with a complex reality and can function as stable dimensions that give meaning to people's lives (see Chapter 4 and 6 about categorization).

Gender Incongruity

Traditional thinking about gender presents a two-gender model in which the child is categorized either as a boy or a girl. Narrow discourses about masculine and feminine gender roles are emphasized from the moment a child enters the world. Gendered codes place the new person within one category and thus communicate from the start (we believe) much about the child and the paths that will lead to a good life that fits what we can see with the naked eye. The child also enters life as a participant

in culture already underway, in which opinions and concepts are negotiated and interpreted (Lock & Strong, 2010). Cultural ways of being,
attitudes and values are woven into the personality through upbringing
and normative expectations of acceptable development. To an extent, the
child is "gendered" through clothes and toys, pronouns, comments and
descriptions. Experience is thus a meaning-creating process, unique to
the individual, but related to the world around us (Grasaasen, 2022).
However, it is here that some children encounter difficulty because they
feel something in themselves that does not resonate with what this world
reflects. Just like culture, nature is diverse and rich in variation and
expression (Coleman et al., 2022).

In society and professional contexts, attitudes show movement towards
normalization and acceptance of gender diversity in human experience,
expression and behaviour as a normal variant of sexual development
(Coleman et al. 2022; Menvielle et al., 2010). The past several decades
have brought new constructions of gender that, simply put, describe fluid
boundaries. These new constructions include transwomen, transmen,
non-binary and gender-rejecting (agender). One of the most significant
developments affecting the quality of life of trans people is the change
in the diagnostic manual of the World Health Organization (WHO;
ICD) of diseases and health-related problems. In ICD-11 approved in
2019, trans-diagnoses were removed and replaced with "gender incongruity". This condition is described as a lack of coherence between
experienced gender or gender identity, and gender assigned at birth. It
also encompasses those who define themselves neither as girl nor boy,
but as having a non-binary gender identity (Coleman et al., 2022). In
earlier ICD manuals, gender incongruence was classified as a psychological illness; now it is described in a chapter on issues and challenges
concerning gender and sexual health. However, it is acknowledged that
gender incongruence can bring discomfort, psychological pain and other
forms of suffering. Related to this new recognition, it has become very
clear how earlier use of terminology has been to categorize and define
gender identities in negative ways. Gender incongruence is not, then,
or now, a psychological illness, and linear explanations have had serious
consequences for people finding themselves within the frame of this
discourse.

When the non-binary came in, there were many who came out. (eepb 2022)

Gender Identity

Some young children, with great clarity and strength of conviction, refer to themselves as having a gender different from that assigned to them by their environment. Other children recognize another gender identity during or after puberty. Often, however, this point of recognition can be traced much farther back than that of self-declaration. For most trans people, gender identity concerns more the desire to move beyond an assigned box than to fit into a new one. Identity can be viewed as the experience of being the same over time, sometimes in contradiction to embodied experience, body image (how we dress and behave) and legal gender (Benestad, 2015). Experience of identity belongs to us as a subjective experience and is a feeling of being unique and independent. Therefore, gender identity has no external reference. It cannot be sensed by others but involves emotional experiences of gender that are not externally measurable. For secure gender identity to be established, others must perceive us as we perceive ourselves (Benestad, 2015; Benestad & Almaas, 2017). Secure gender belonging requires compliance between subjective experience of gender and its positive confirmation by our environment. Self-knowledge arises through interaction and relationship. We contribute continually to one another's emerging identities and only become real living people when we are included through this interaction in a social world of significance and as part of society at large (Dallos & Draper, 2015).

Our understandings of phenomena are characterized by cultural themes. Constraints in the form of meta-narratives set the conditions that determine the stories that get highlighted and those that remain in the dark. Often narratives of what is usual are accommodated while those about what is more seldom are disavowed (Grasaasen, 2022). When a breach arises between the narrative images children and youth have of themselves and those they receive from their surroundings, they may attempt to resolve this by striving towards preferred cultural descriptions, driven by feelings of deviance and abnormality. Many children and youth do not feel at home in the external culture or in their own immediate environments because what they are unable to provide what is demanded of them. Difficulties in construction of a secure self-image and good quality of life therefore does not primarily concern their own gender experience but is shaped by the preconceptions of their surroundings and by social discrimination. The feeling of differentness can lead to lack of belonging and the feeling of outsider-ship. This can be understood from several perspectives. Adolescence is a vulnerable period in which development is learned in relationship with others. Youth travel in groups, arm-in-arm. At the same time, research shows that verbal harassment occurs frequently among adolescents, usually in the form of gendered words with negative connotations and steeped in traditional gender roles. The perceptions youth have of themselves are thus partially the result of linguistic and relational experiences (Grasaasen, 2019). However, these words also pull towards limited categories and block perception of different descriptions lying outside of these. Experiences leave traces. Research shows how children and youth with different gender affiliation who experience bullying can develop psychological problems, indulge in self-harm and substance abuse and have an increased risk of suicide (Eisenberg et al., 2017; Gower et al., 2018).

It is a consequence in itself, that offensive words and expressions follow a traditional gender pattern that helps to maintain prejudices and stigmatizing attitudes. However, we wish to make clear that youth have their experiences along marked paths (Grasaasen, 2019). In a discursive perspective, gender and sexuality are not givens, nor stable, consistent quantities, but linguistic, appearing through historical, social and institutional practices (Foucault, 1998).

Family and Parenthood

Discourses of gender affect behaviour and development, mostly perhaps in relation to family relationships. Familial roles such as mother/ father, daughter/son, brother/ sister and grandmother/grandfather are also delineated along gender-binary axes and come with sets of expectations for role performance. The family is a strong discourse founded on the idea that, despite its many and modern forms, it will remain important throughout life. It is the smallest, most fundamental and intimate context of life as well as a significant social institution. For most people, it will have great relational value from birth to death. The family creates a safe base for protection, development and learning in childhood—throughout the teen years and for many, throughout the lifespan. There are exceptions of course, but in crucial life phases and in life crises, it is those we view as our closest family who primarily and to the greatest extent are involved. When children and youth experience differentness, family support has been shown to function as a protective factor against negative consequences such as psychological problems and substance abuse (Gower et al., 2018).

Most parents want the best for their children and for them to have a good childhood and grow up to be independent adults with rewarding lives. However, parenthood is also discursively governed and strict norms exist for how best to perform it and what this should involve. Like the family, parenthood is a cultural construction undergoing continuous change. Recent decades have seen development of a discourse of "intensive parenthood" (Hays, 1998), in which children's needs come first and significant time, energy and material resources are dedicated to their upbringing (Faircloth, 2014). The modern relationship between parents and children is largely borne through emotional bonds and independent of the extended family. Modern parenthood can be viewed as a relational project in which discourses of love define parent-child interaction in the family. The emphasis on care is also an expression of love and makes it visible. Parenthood is experienced as meaningful because of love and the parental role has personal value as a meaningful task. The cultural expectation of placing the child at the centre is the foundation for the practice of "child-led response" when children and youth show gender incongruity (Edwards-Leeper et al., 2016). Many parents express how their unconditional love for their child overrides a divergent gender identity. However, this also involves practical and emotional challenges for parents, siblings and close others (Wahlig, 2015). The family as a system is greater than itself; it is a composite of all the ideas, dreams, significances and expectations of its members and of one another. Parental decisions about how to support one another, also when this becomes difficult, will therefore be influenced by the implicit backdrop of cultural constructions of what it means to be a family and of good parenthood. It is from within this picture that some parents react strongly when their children "come out". Parents can feel a sense of loss and confusion around their child's new identity and role in the family. Many wonder how they will be treated by others and how life will be from now on. For some, this initiates a significant grief process. Parents describe also grieving the loss of family identity, especially if the child changes their first name, which usually has special meaning. They may also grieve over loss of the familial past, over how their child's gender-related experience has not been authentic (Wahlig, 2015).

Some parents spend significant time finding out how to move from shock and grief through resistance to acceptance. Even though they want the best for their child, not all believe that a different gender path is the correct one. They can be afraid their child will be bullied or excluded. Some parents also have criticisms of a religious or political nature, or they have a value system that creates resistance (Zamboni, 2006). Other parents find it easier to support the child's experience and development. They feel pride in the child who has the strength and courage to be seen, and they may experience a stronger bond to the child and within the family (Gonzalez et al., 2013). Family support is not, however, a one-dimensional or simple process, and stigma and marginalization within the environment will affect everyone in the family (Menvielle & Hill, 2010). All family members have their own processes to move through before they "come out" as siblings, parents or grandparents of a trans person. In addition, it can be stressful to have such a significant focus on the family system, and this may change relationships between members. This can result in changed relational attachment and poorer family function over shorter or longer periods (Westwater et al., 2019).

An Inclusive Conversational Space

Welcome!

Offering an inclusive environment in which youth, parents and significant others can feel welcome, confirmed and seen is the prerequisite for family therapy to make a difference. The alliance can only be established if the relationship is experienced as equal and the conversational space a safe place for exploration. Non-verbal communication begins before the conversation starts. Use of context markers in the space enables us to declare awareness, interest and experience. These can be pictures, a pride flag or literature that indicate implicitly where we stand as safe conversational partners. Further, as systemic therapists, we are guests in their lives and should be respectful, informed by our knowledge of marginalization and social debate. Which pronoun do they want us to use? Her, hen, him, they, them, ze or perhaps a preferred name?

As family therapists we must also care for those around the child or youth, and it is important for a good exploratory process that therapists act as hopeful supporters for all involved. Parents can feel guilt and low self-confidence as parents. Therefore, we require knowledge of parental experiences when children are different; it is also imperative to understand what makes the family a good place to be throughout the exploration of the child's gender identity (Wahlig, 2015). Other essential knowledge includes that of trans identities and a base understanding of central concepts of significance for conversations about gender. In this way, we avoid having to question children, youth and parents and prevent them from feeling that they must teach the therapist or explain themselves in an intimate way. We must help to locate hope and coping strategies that can make the future manageable. Knowing the terminology is the key to being able to confirm experiences and feelings, expand understanding and build bridges between people and ideas.

As therapists, we must not forget that we are also part of a family, a society and a culture and remain self-reflexively aware of our own constructions. We must continually reflect over our understanding of what we read in the social and academic debates and actively assess the extent to which these discourses interfere with our curiosity and ability to wonder. Our preconceptions usually lie implicitly as a confusing back-drop the effect of which is difficult to control. Before reflection can begin, it has already taken up a place, and we draw our prejudices with us into the professional conversation (Grasaasen, 2022). We must never believe that we know how another's lifeworld is, but as far as possible take responsibility for remaining open to what the other needs.

The Conversations: Include All the Significant Others You Want

Usually, children and youth arrive at conversations with at least one parent, sometimes also with a sibling or grandparent. There is a saying that it takes a village to raise a child. Our slogan is include as many as you want among meaningful others. The entire system around a child is significant because all people need to experience belongingness to others to have a good life. The family is a system also surrounded by other systems of significance for the change process. For children and youth, these will include relatives, friends, teachers and other important persons from school and free time activities. They can act as buffers in meetings with challenges and be supporters of healthy development (Benestad, 2015; Benestad & Almaas, 2017; Eisenberg et al., 2017).

We have arranged with Sarah to speak with Mum and Dad without her present.

Mum: Sarah has always been a bit special, but lately everything's gotten so difficult. She says that she's a boy. I just can't believe that. I don't understand it. What kind of an idea is that? That's why we got in touch because I don't believe in this thing about changing gender. I think she's depressed and needs someone to talk to.

Just as strongly as we hear the despair in Sarah's voice, we can hear it now in a grieving mother. Dad says little but shows his support with small gestures while Mum speaks. We acknowledge them for having sought help and emphasize the courage this takes. Being a parent is personal and private, and a role we like to believe we master. I ask if we can talk a little about Sarah in relation to what she experiences and says. When they think back on Sarah's childhood and upbringing, how was she as a child?

Mum: I don't know what to say. I've got so many questions, but so few answers. Sarah has always been different from her sister, but they've been good friends and I know her sister has defended her when others have called her odd. As we're talking now, I feel mostly how afraid I am for her. Children can be so nasty. What if she gets bullied? How will her life be now? What if we put in motion something she'll regret? What if she won't be able to have kids?

In describing how conversations with families about gender incongruence can be conducted, it is reductionistic to retell only one narrative in a landscape that is so multifaceted and dominated by tabus, resistance, denial, secrecy and shame. This is true especially for the child or youth, but also for parents and siblings who find gender incongruence difficult to understand and manage. Sarah and her parents can nevertheless illustrate the ambiguity that often appears, but which also makes gender incongruence possible to grasp and to talk about. On the reverse side of love, we find dread of not being enough, grief over losing the child they thought they had and fear of the unknown.

When families seek help, this may be because the situation has become so stuck that constructive communication has become impossible, more often, however, they seek guidance and support to assist the child- or adolescents process towards belongingness. Facilitating family conversations thus involves creating a direction in which all participants come into position to speak and listen to one another. Sometimes, it may be necessary to have conversations with family members on their own. Parents and others who feel guilt can benefit from opportunities to express uncertainty, grief and discomfort without their child or youth present. Just as important is having one-to-one conversations with the child or youth. The goal of the conversation is to support the child's exploration such that they can feel secure and self-sufficient using their own expressions, standing on their own two feet. The reactions of parents and close others will influence how the child or youth thinks about themselves. Parents are usually the first to experience the child's attempts to create agreement between inner and outer self-images. They also have some power to determine the extent to which the child or youth is allowed to express their gender identity through clothing, pronouns and name. Denial from them can limit space for action and make the child invisible. Further, the child can turn frustration inward and blame themselves for their differentness (Eisenberg et al., 2017).

> I hear Mum's uncertainty about how to handle Sarah's experiences and how to think about the future. I ask how they as parents talk about this at home?

> Dad: It's difficult because we think quite differently. I'm also worried about Sarah, but right now I can't get concerned about her adult life or what other people think. I want her to feel better right now. What can I do for her? She's a fantastic child having a hard time. I agree that she's always been different, but I've been a bit proud of that, and thought that it's sort of cool to have a child who's so independent and unconcerned with being like everyone else. At the same time, I understand that this must have cost Sarah more than what I've understood, and I feel guilty for overlooking what she's tried to tell us. I wonder what she thinks about me. As her dad, I should probably have known her as well as she knows herself?

> To generalize, I choose to conventionalize his question (Bruner, 2003) as reflecting ideas he probably shares with many other parents of children the same age. I refer to Sarah's independence as well. In what way has he contributed to this quality Sarah is certainly happy to have now?

In gender incongruence, family support has been shown to be particularly protective of psychological health of children and youth (Abreu et al., 2022). Unfortunately, it also happens that parents refuse to acknowledge their child's gender identity and the family becomes divided. Occasionally, we see that youth break with those closest to them to establish themselves in another family or within a network in which they can feel at home. It is then even more important for the therapist to acknowledge the unique needs of the youth and act as an allied party (Eisenberg, 2017).

From Different to Talented

The power of language becomes extra clear when those we speak with have marginal voices (Moscheta & Rasera, 2021). When children and families feel excluded and different, the use of inclusive language can make a big difference. The goal of professional conversations is to create change. We must, therefore, inspire by being unprejudiced and resourceful and use the language of co-creative action. We must speak in a way that gives hope, pride, meaning and movement towards the new and better. Maturana and Varela (1987) describe three fundamental elements that together and reciprocally stimulate opportunities for growth, development and change: love, external guidance and time for reflection. Therapists can support the family by investigating, deconstructing and reshaping cultural and familial discourses around gender and transgender identities. Through reflective processes, we can actively search out several perspectives, new understandings and other ways of communicating.

> Sarah is lucky. In their own individual ways, Mum and Dad talk about great love for a loved child. She has one parent most concerned about what is happening now, while the other is thinking about the future. Together, this yields a difference that is both complementary, double and provides space for two thoughts at the same time. What do they think when I summarize what they have said in this way?
>
> Mum: That sounds much better but it's difficult as well because it continues to give us different roles. Dad as always, is the nice one and understanding, while I'm the difficult one asking questions. We need to learn to talk about this in a way that makes Sarah understand that we're cooperating, and that we're afraid of doing something now that might be wrong later on.

Connotations have significant place in systemic conversations and can be defined as the meaning a word or action receives through how it is coloured or presented with a positive or negative nuance. Positive connotation is an active reformulation in which we seek ways to give words and phenomena additional, attractive meaning. This is an active change of awareness and a skill the therapist can employ to show the significance complexity and avoid oversimplified and linear descriptions. When we bring a positive connotation to the negative this puts Yin and Yang together to form a whole (Hoffman, 1981). As an example, we raise the expression, "born in the wrong body", one Sarah uses about herself. The expression has become widespread among those it describes, in the media and in public discussions. It is used as a personal narrative, a description of other people's experience, and by health professionals speaking about gender incongruence. As a metaphor it has temporary meaning but for several reasons, we do not find the expressions well-connoted. Firstly, no one is born in the wrong body because no body is wrong. Secondly, no one can exchange their body for another, and if Sarah had been born in another body, she would have been someone else. On the contrary, we can believe that people are born with different talents, also for gender. We can positively connote a youth's experiences and call this trans talent or talent for gender (Benestad & Almaas, 2017). It will also make a big difference in conversations with Sarah and her parents if instead of describing her as *odd and different*, she is called *courageous and talented*. The goal can also be to get the parents to place Sarah's experience into a framework that is easier to relate to. Movement towards a more appropriate understanding can occur if the conversation can be led towards resources over faults and deficiencies. In the same way, we can construe the term "trans-aesthetic" to make it easier for all to see the beautiful in the androgynous.

Gender Map

The gender map is a therapeutic and educational tool developed by Silje-Håvard Bolstad (2019), based on a way of thinking about gender developed by Almaas and Benestad (2017). It is a visual picture that can be used as an aid in conversations with slightly older children, youth, adults, parents and networks. The idea is that it is open and only roughly refers to categories of gender without presenting uniform answers. We find it of great usefulness, not least because it provides children and youth with a seamless opportunity to set their own "brand" on the map and enable them to move it again at a later point. This permits reflection over feelings and experiences they have had, before and now, related to development and age. Defining gender as fluid means that the idea of who one is can change over time and that is fine. An important feature of map use is that gender is not thought of in terms of opposites. The opposite of a girl is not a boy, but a non-girl, and a boy is not the opposite of a girl, but non-boy (Fig. 3.1).

The farther to the right a child or youth moves on the map, in every vertical axis is the extent to which they feel like a girl and the farther up along all horizontal axes, the extent to which they feel like a boy. This means that in the right-hand corner they feel both very girl and very boy—an example of the non-binary experience. Feeling a pure girl identity or pure boy identity is an experience of finding oneself, respectively, in the lower right and upper left corners. There are few children and youth who place themselves in the one-dimensional corners, and those

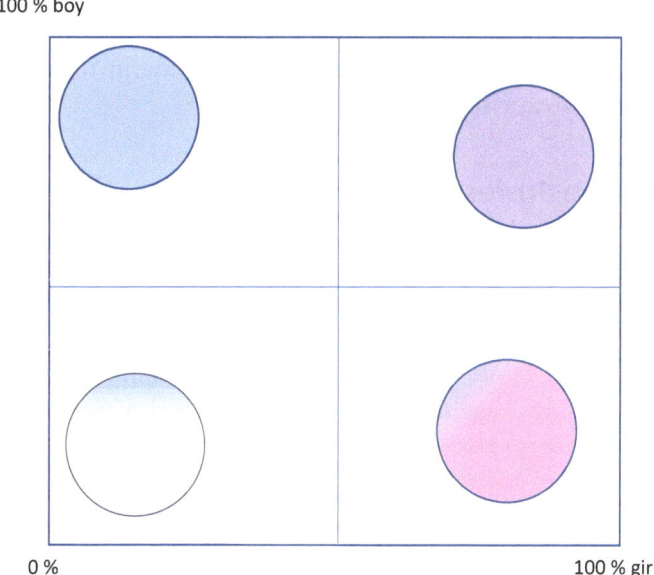

Fig. 3.1 Gender map (reproduced by the authors, based on Bolstad, 2019) (www.gendermap.no)

who do are often on a desperate hunt to be their experienced gender. They experience themselves as binary and find their place in the upper right portion of the map or in the lower left portion. Close by these placements we usually find those who experience themselves either as transwomen or transmen. Down in the left corner, a youth has no experience of being a gender, a different, but also non-binary experience. Those who place themselves here have the greatest challenges, because as a society, we still find it difficult to find space for such (gender) expression. In this context, we see constructions of types of dress, makeup and beards.

There is a wide space outside the binary boxes, and this provides the opportunity to locate oneself in multiple places, wherever one wishes along the spectrum. Those who find their place in the map often want to alter their lives, outward appearance and sometimes their bodies to harmonize as well as possible with their gender identities. The map can also open to conversations about narrow discourses of masculinity and femininity to expand the image of what is common. In this way, we can be challenged to think in new ways about narrow gender roles and what is required for children and youth to feel at home in themselves, with the gender they experience.

An Inclusive Professional Community

While changes are occurring that reveal more inclusive images of children, youth and gender incongruity, we continue to inhabit a professional landscape with divergent opinions and significant disagreement. The power of academic positions is still used to promote some ideas and suppress others in ways that create division. This in turn affects development of and opportunities for locating help. Along with a sharpened social debate this can alienate those children, youth and parents experiencing gender incongruity seeking acknowledgement of their needs. Within a social constructionist perspective, we view previous practice as a collective construction in which most recognized knowledge has been shaped within a categorizing and discriminative tradition (Moscheta & Rasera, 2021). We believe that a relational and social constructionist approach to family conversations can be helpful and make a difference. We also believe in dialogue and in the opportunities that can appear if we seek a multiverse in which opinions produce expansion instead of restriction. Then we can address the importance of the power and influence of the environment, acknowledge the rights of all children and youth to live in a healthy milieu, turn narratives of difference around and promote what is beautiful on the other side of difficult experiences.

References

Abreu, P. D., Andrade, R. L. D. P., Maza, I. L. D. S., Faria, M. G. B. F. D., Nogueira, J. D. A., & Monroe, A. A. (2022). Dynamics of primary social networks to support mothers, fathers, or guardians of transgender children and adolescents: A systematic review. *Public Health, 19*, 7941. https://doi.org/10.3390/ijerph19137941

Almaas, E., & Benestad, E. E. P. (2017). *Sexologi i praksis [Sexology in practice]*. Universitetsforlaget.

Andersen, N., & Malterud, K. (2013). *Seksuell orientering og levekår [Sexual orientation and living conditions]*. Uni Helse.

Benestad, E. E. P. (2015). Gender belonging. Children, adolescents, adults and the role of the therapist. *The International Journal of Narrative Therapy and Community Work, 2016*(4).

Bolstad, S.-H. (2019). Gender map. Downloaded 1.5.23 from https://www.gendermap.no

Bruner, J. (2003). *Making stories: Law, literature, life*. Harvard University Press.

Butler, C., Beavis, J., Aldallal, F., Nelson-Hall, S., & Shah-Beckley, I. (2022). The social construction of gender variance in childhood, adolescence and parenthood: A story completion study. *Journal of Family Therapy, 44*, 264–278. https://doi.org/10.1111/1467-6427.12348

Butler, C. (2018). The social construction of non-binary gender identity. *Context, 155*, 27–30.

Coleman A. E., Radix, A. E., Bouman, W. P., Brown, G. R., De Vries, A. L., Deutsch, M. B., Ettner, R., Fraser, L., Goodman, M., Green, J., & Hancock, A. B. (2022). Standards of care for the health of transgender and gender diverse people, Version 8. *International Journal of Transgender Health, 6*(23 (Suppl 1)), S1–S259. https://doi.org/10.1080/26895269.2022.2100644

Dallos, R., & Draper, R. (2015). *An introduction to family therapy*. Open University Press.

Edwards-Leeper, L., Leibowitz, S., & Sangganjanavanich, V. F. (2016). Affirmative practice with transgender and gender nonconforming youth: Expanding the model. *Psychology of Sexual Orientation and Gender Diversity, 3*(2). https://doi.org/10.1037/sgd0000167

Eisenberg, M. E., Gower, A. L., McMorris, B. J., Rider, G. N., Shea, G., & Coleman, E. (2017, October). Risk and protective factors in the lives of transgender/gender non-conforming adolescents. *Adolescent Health, 61*(4), 521–526. https://doi.org/10.1016/j.jadohealth.2017.04.014

Faircloth, C. (2014). Intensive parenting and the expansion of parenting. In E. Lee, J. Bristow, C. Faircloth, & J. Macvarish (Eds.), *Parenting culture studies* (pp. 25–50). Palgrave Macmillan.

Foucault, M. (1998). *The will to knowledge. The history of sexuality*. Penguin Books Ltd.

Gonzalez, K. A., Rostosky, S. S., Odom, R. D., & Riggle, E. D. B. (2013). The positive aspects of being the parent of an LGBTQ child. *Family Process, 52*(2), 325–337. https://doi.org/10.1111/famp.12009

Gower, A. L., Rider, G. N., Brown, C., McMorris, B. J., Coleman, E., Taliaferro, L. A., & Eisenberg, M. E. (2018). Supporting transgender and gender diverse youth: Protection against emotional distress and substance use. *American Journal of Preventive Medicine., 55*(6), 787–794. https://doi.org/10.1016/j.amepre.2018.06.030

Grasaasen, A. (2019). "It's just something we say". A narrative overview of literature on the consequences of the youth phenomenon of verbal sexual harassment. *Fokus på Familien, 3*, 217–237. Universitetsforlaget.

Grasaasen, A. (2022). My mother, my mirror? Three generations encounter family therapy. *Journal of Family Therapy, 44*(4), 462–473. https://doi.org/10.1111/1467-6427.12413

Hays, S. (1998). *Cultural contradictions of motherhood*. Yale University Press.

Hoffman, I. (1981). *Foundation of family therapy; a conceptual framework for systems changes*. Basic Books.

Lock, A., & Strong, T. (2010). *Social constructionism: Sources and stirrings in theory and practice*. Cambridge University Press.

Maturana, H. R., & Varela, F. J. (1987). *The tree of knowledge*. New Science Library.

Menvielle, E. M. D., Darryl B., & Hill, D. B. (PhD). (2010). An affirmative intervention for families with gender-variant children: A process evaluation.

Journal of Gay & Lesbian Mental Health, 15(1), 94–123.https://doi.org/10.1080/19359705.2011.530576

Moscheta, M. S., & Rasera, E. F. (2021). *Health care practices for LGBT people.* (Red) McNamee, S., Gergen, M., Camargo-Borges, C., Rasera, E. F. *Social constructionist practice.* SAGE Publications Ltd.

Wahlig, J. L. (2015). Losing the child they thought they had: Therapeutic suggestions for an ambiguous loss perspective with parents of a transgender child. *Journal of GLBT Family Studies, 11*(4), 305–326. https://doi.org/10.1080/1550428X.2014.945676

Westwater, J. J., Riley, E. A., & Peterson, G. M. (2019). What about the family in youth gender diversity? A literature review. *International Journal of Transgenderism, 20*(4), 351–370. https://doi.org/10.1080/15532739.2019.1652130

Zamboni, B. D. (2006). Therapeutic considerations in working with the family, friends, and partners of transgendered individuals. *Family Journal, 14*(2), 174–179. https://doi.org/10.1177/1066480705285251

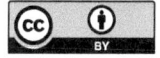

4

Relational Interventions in Complex Situations: Sessions with Substance Using Parents

Siv Merete Myra

Hanne is afraid of losing her three-month-old daughter Ina. Hanne has used substances since the age of twelve. She and her boyfriend Martin, who is Ina's father, have been in the family unit of a substance use facility for almost eight months. Hanne is worried about her relationship to Martin and his substance use problems. The parents need help for their substance use problems, as well as help to be good enough parents for Ina.

> Hanne said: "We need help to be a normal family without substance use".
> Martin said: "I'm afraid society has already condemned us".

Their words and worries stuck with me. How could we help this family get back to society? They felt misunderstood and were afraid of the child protection services.

S. M. Myra (✉)
Department of Family Therapy and Systemic Practice, Faculty of Social Studies, VID Specialized University, Oslo, Norway
e-mail: siv.merete.myra@vid.no

© The Author(s) 2024
S. M. Myra et al. (eds.), *New Horizons in Systemic Practice with Children and Families*, Palgrave Texts in Counselling and Psychotherapy,
https://doi.org/10.1007/978-3-031-38111-9_4

This chapter describes therapeutic encounters with Hanne 28, Martin 30 and their three-month-old daughter Ina. The parents have substance use problems and are undergoing treatment in an inpatient family unit in a Norwegian specialist healthcare facility. Case-based illustrations are used to describe the couple's dilemmas. New horizons in this chapter will try to illustrate that it can be easy to lose sight of how a small intervention can be big enough in the first sessions with the parents.

Essential Elements in the Meetings with Hanne and Martin

A systemic approach was used to describe the sessions with the parents. A systemic and relational approach is rooted in a social constructionist understanding (Lock & Strong, 2014). In order to meet the needs of these families, it is important to gain an understanding of what they themselves describe as their difficulties. The parents' experiences and dilemmas are often linked to their feelings of lack of recognition, low self-esteem and their doubts about whether they can be good enough parents (Aamodt, 2009). The therapists, for their part, want to provide the best treatment. The question of whether contextual factors and a focus on psychological resources dominate in counselling sessions can be influenced by circulating discourses about what is good parenting. One dominant discourse within the field, in addition to the social and cultural discourses, concerns the importance of making efforts to improve harmony and attachment between parents and children (Myra et al., 2018). One dilemma is that a strong focus on improving parenting can overshadow efforts to solve the parental addiction problems.

In clinical practice, therapists have been confronted with the challenge of discourses about how generational cycles of abuse can prevent the development of secure attachment and positive interaction with children (Myra et al., 2018; Wiig et al., 2018). A further dominant argument has been that parents with substance use problems will find it difficult to both adopt and understand their children's perspective, as their attention is drawn towards their craving for alcohol or drugs (Søderstrøm &

Skårderud, 2009). Research by Wiig et al. (2018) reveals that therapists are often in a dilemma. Parents who themselves have experienced substance use in their homes faced many challenges. Therapists found it very challenging to conduct sessions with parents with young children in cases of intergenerational substance use because the dilemma described by the therapists involved a desire to rescue the child in contrast to treating the parents. The therapists wanted to give parents and children a good start, even though it could turn out that the parents' care was assessed as inadequate. The element of hope in this approach was the knowledge that having a child could also represent a window of opportunity for change and motivation to cease substance use, which was an optimistic and potent factor in sessions with these families (Wiig et al., 2018). In a systemic approach, the therapist will focus on achieving a new level of knowledge by raising awareness of how Hanne and Martin affect and are affected by context and relationships (Lock & Strong, 2014).

In the counselling sessions with Hanne and Martin, a narrative approach was also used. The aim of this was to search for new meaning by expanding the understanding of the stories they shared. Their challenges and dilemmas are presented as small stories that describe what they find difficult. By creating a story that incorporates the past, the present and thoughts about the future, new narratives can be generated. By asking questions such as "What do you want your future life to be like?", the context can be explored, and alternative stories can be created (White & Epston, 1990). The sessions with this family involved an exploration of themes around addiction, parenting and ideas about how we should live our lives.

In a systemic approach, and as part of the method of counselling clients, we can explore the prevailing discourses in greater detail. Discourses point to established truths in society. Discourses can lead to social practices and expectations and show how social meaning and structure are constructed in a professional, social and cultural context (Lock & Strong, 2014; White, 1984).

A clinical context enables the sharing and processing of painful stories that are often "stuck". By using a narrative approach, we can together create new stories and challenge established discourses. In the sessions with Hanne and Martin, the aim was to create new understanding, a new experience of meaning and new hope. An understanding of experiences passed down through generations, and of the fact that we are shaped by nature and nurture, our environment and contextual experiences can all be appreciated and reflected on in a relational perspective (Andersen, 2011; Gergen, 2010). In terms of therapy, this is also a question of a shift from a psychodynamic focus on intrapsychic conflicts to a perspective that deals with interpersonal relationships. In modern attachment theory, the understanding is that different types of attachment behaviour in adulthood will be based on subjective childhood experiences, but also influenced by the specific context. Attachment may thus be understood as a result of both early attachment history and current circumstances (Bowlby, 1998). This can be important knowledge for therapists in interaction with clients such as Hanne and Martin when they describe family substance use problems in their own childhood. In summary, findings from a number of studies show how adverse childhood experiences such as parental substance abuse can disrupt a child's normal development (Felitti & Anda, 2010).

The Background and Context of Therapy for Parents of Young Children

Substance use and parenting are often two competing systems: research shows that the neurological pathways involved in substance use are the same as those involved in parenting capacity (Reading, 2002). This explains why children "compete" with alcohol or drugs for their parents' attention. Substance use treatment from a family perspective thus involves reinstating the parenting capacity by preventing the competing use. This includes promoting the parents' emotional availability and capacity for action, and one explanation is that attachment to one's child involves both an emotional relationship and an action-oriented perspective (Stern, 2004).

Parental substance use is often a complex problem; Hanne and Martin grew up with substance use and socio-economic challenges in their homes and also in addition to poor, vulnerable social networks that had provided little support. In clinical practice, therapists have been confronted with the challenge of discourses about how generational cycles of abuse can prevent attachment and positive interaction with children (Myra et al., 2018; Wiig et al., 2018).

Examples of Dialogues and Topics

New Horizons—Small Interventions in Complex Situations

Counselling sessions with parents often deal with what the parents themselves introduce as their perceived dilemmas or challenges. Exploring Hanne and Martin's context involves not only exploring dilemmas linked to the topics raised but also perspectives such as being aware of dilemmas between these topics and the encounter with the therapist. One such dilemma can be the therapist's feeling of being caught between professional, social and cultural norms and discourses. A systemic approach implies understanding of how we have a relational influence on each other. This means that we are not only concerned with the topic as such, but also with exploring the relationship between the therapist and the parents, and thus the effects of the relational element. Relevant questions may then focus on *how* to create a therapeutic space that helps the parents to open up, and *how* to create a relationship that influences co-creation in the encounter. Common factors such as trust, hope and faith are vital to family counselling. By adopting a systemic approach, we see contextual constraints rather than individual shortcomings. Understanding addiction involves a realization that it is a complex matter, requiring slow processes and small interventions where the focus should be on creating a context for a resource-based and relational perspective. In this way, a systemic perspective is put to work through the understanding that we influence and are influenced by each other in interaction and dialogue. Exploring together and involving various perspectives can lead to change (Andersen, 2011).

The therapist's position in the counselling session may be a "not-knowing stance"; this means that we could not know or make any statement about the other's experiences until we had asked for and listened to the story told by Hanne and Martin (Anderson, 2003). In this approach, showing interest and respect for the other person's story is crucial to establishing a dialogue. The therapist *does have* knowledge in terms of asking new questions, having opinions, speculations or suggestions. The therapist asks for permission to share knowledge, through a story, questions, comments, suggestions and reflection and also anticipates perspectives that differ from the initial questions she brought to the encounter (Andersen, 2005).

I will now describe some more sequences from the sessions with Hanne and Martin. Here, I will attempt to show how the knowledge we have about the relationship between attachment experiences, intergenerational processes and contextual factors can be reflected in their therapy. I will then describe what is important to me as a therapist and try to show how I connect to Hanne and Martin, as individuals, as a couple and as parents. The context will be an attempt to establish trust and safety, a context for exploration and dialogue.

The parents were asked to express their expectations and wishes. *Hanne said: "I'm so afraid the child welfare people will take Ina away, so that we, the parents, won't get a chance to show we can do good enough parenting".*

Here, Hanne sheds light on her feeling of a lack of trust and recognition for their situation as parents, and her fear that there will be little discussion of contextual factors. The relevant issue here was how the therapist could create a therapeutic space that helped the parents to open up. In my conversations with Hanne and Martin, I focused on exploring contextual constraints such as socio-economic factors, rather than individual shortcomings and psychological capacity. The goal was to create safety in small steps and try to create a base of security.

Martin said: "I feel the system has already condemned us". This statement illustrates the importance of taking the time to listen to parents' feelings and descriptions. How could I as a therapist create a space that invited Hanne and Martin to gain enough confidence to see for themselves what their challenges were and how could this reduce their feeling of being stigmatized?

Hanne said: "We've suffered so much, I don't trust anyone, and I'm afraid to say what I really feel".

Martin said: "The system doesn't think we can be good parents because of our baggage in life. They think that because we grew up with substance abuse and suffered a lot, we don't know how to be good parents for Ina".

Another approach illustrated by the counselling sessions was Bakhtin's (1981) concept of polyphony, where the different voices of Hanne, Martin and the therapist were shared.

Hanne said: That when I heard Martins concern about "losing" Ina, it awakened a fighting spirit in me. Here, we can see that the feeling of a fighting spirit creates hope, hope that they as parents could be able to bring about change in their life.

This concept helps us to understand how a plurality of voices emerges, creating new understanding by bringing in more voices. Allowing more voices to be heard presents more aspects of the phenomenon and provides more possibilities to address the perceived complexity of the situation. In a narrative approach, the opportunity to tell and retell, as well as to listen to different perspectives, will provide the freedom to develop one's own understanding of the challenges revealed in the narratives and to talk about them in new ways (White, 1984).

When Are Small Interventions Big Enough?

Before describing more statements with these parents, I would like to mention some topics that typically arise in the family units of specialist healthcare facilities when the parents have both substances use problems and young children. At such treatment facilities, typical topics are the parents' awareness of parenting and addiction, and also in many cases the understanding of how generational adverse experiences can affect internal working models of attachment and one's own parenting style. Parents are often the bearers of a complex set of problems, which can make it difficult for therapists to decide what they should focus on in their work, and what they believe is feasible in terms of achieving good enough parenting. It is therefore necessary to be aware of the importance of creating a working alliance between therapist and Hanne and Martin that helps to develop emotional organization based on trust, respect and mutual recognition. When working with these families, it can be easy to lose sight of how a small intervention can be big enough in the first sessions with the parents. "Big enough" in the early stages can be to attempt to create a space where the parents feel sufficiently safe to dare to share something of themselves. Awareness of common factors such as trust, hope and faith can help to co-create a relationship that can influence the working model. In encounters with these families, the important factor may be belief in bringing about change, which may require a systemic approach that considers contextual constraints rather than individual shortcomings.

Martin said; when I listened to Hanne talk about how she felt a fighting spirit, my fatherly feelings awakened, and I felt that I as a father would fight like a soldier for my family. Here, we can see how an overall perspective can involve an approach where the counselling sessions focus on co-creating new narratives and an orientation towards resources and mastery. Thus, the power that lies in the verification of the narrative, including by the listeners, becomes a key element of this working model (Johnsen & Torsteinsson, 2012).

When talking to Hanne and Martin, the aim was to open up new perspectives. A narrative approach allowed us to see that it was not just a question of psychological resources and one's own childhood experiences, but the possibility of positioning oneself to explore elements of contextual factors. By eliciting Hanne and Martin's descriptions through telling new stories, we could bring out what they wanted to achieve. When the parents shared their narrative and received help to obtain more voices than the "stuck" voice, a new understanding with more perspectives was created. Hanne said, that when she heard Martin's concern about "losing" Ina, it awakened a fighting spirit in her, and a hope that they as parents will be able to bring about changes in their lives. Martin said, when he listened to Hanne talk about how she felt a fighting spirit, his fatherly feelings awakened, he felt that he as a father would fight like a soldier for his family.

Seeing a dilemma from different angles also enables us to see alternatives and alternative identities and thus new perspectives. When the parents were able to tell and retell, and listen to each other, the narrative changed from hopelessness to the belief in becoming good enough parents for Ina. By creating a space that helps clients open up, the therapist will also have to be open to seeing her practice in a new light. This could mean becoming aware of her prejudices and her own dilemmas, as well as the influence of prevailing professional, social and cultural discourses, which will enable her to talk to parents in new ways (Myra, 2017).

By adopting a dialogic and reflexive approach in counselling sessions with parents, one can explore topics relevant to the parents' dilemmas. The attempt to create a relationship that affects their working models raises questions such as: How can Hanne and Martin be invited to understandings that provide safety and reduce stigma? A self-reflexive approach will focus on interaction and relationships, which also enables the therapist to think through her actions, prejudices and reactions, leading to greater reflection and self-awareness. Another aspect of this approach is increased awareness of the possible effect of family life and cultural context on professional practice (Vetere & Stratton, 2016).

Two questions that arose in the sessions with Hanne and Martin were *how* to make it easier for the therapist to explore their way of understanding on the parents' own terms, and *how* to talk to them to prevent them from feeling that their own inadequacies are the key issue, rather than external factors and circumstances in their lives. If this could be achieved, it would hopefully reduce the parents' feeling of being stigmatized. The aim would be for Hanne and Martin to gain sufficient trust to prevent them from adapting their narratives and perceived stigma to cultural norms and people's expectations of them, but instead to dare to share something of themselves. The attempt to create a reflexive space to explore the complexity, without any blueprint for success, was a useful perspective in the sessions with the couple.

Enabling a dialogic process in the sessions where everyone is allowed to speak avoids having to find a solution to the problem too soon. This approach offers a way of working together that involves asking exploratory questions about how far things make sense and how this may change over time. For example, the exploration in the sessions with Hanne and Martin involved underlining how relationships are in themselves interactions and how challenges are not merely psychological but can also be created through relationships. If we did not include the relational perspective, we might, in the worst case, maintain and reinforce the stigma they already perceived as pervading their lives. The challenge for the therapist may be to take the time to let Hanne and Martin tell their stories for themselves. Here, key questions were *how* to position oneself to help the parents share something of themselves, and *what would happen* if the parents felt safe enough to share their challenges in this way, without adapting to norms and stigma? The narrative tradition uses externalization, in this way the substance use problem becomes something other than themselves; it becomes an extraneous element that they need help to explore. By externalizing the problem, one avoids the potential constraining effects of the professional, social and cultural discourses. If addiction is excluded from the parents' identity, it becomes easier to form an opinion on and counteract it. Including the perspective of hope with therapeutic perspectives can create a resilient context, build bridges and provide a space where parents can gain new relational experiences. Bordin (1994) describes a working alliance as involving emotional organization based on trust, respect and mutual recognition. If parents feel safe enough to think about what affects parenting, they may ask themselves: *What effect do my previous experiences have on my ability to be a good parent?* If there are no significant others to support the parents, counselling sessions will be a vital intervention. A focus on change in internal working models in these sessions will add new and changed relational experiences. The parent-child relationship can then change from reactive to reflective parenting (Stern, 2004). This involves interaction and an emphasis on intersubjective processes in an interplay with therapeutic techniques. It could also involve creating a space where the therapist-client relationship enables the experience of new ways of feeling safe in relation to others. This can be described as tuning in and resonance; the therapist tunes in to Hanne's and Martin's own ideas and focuses on the signals they provide, while still being conscious of her own ideas and stigma. Resonance or the experience of being held, by being seen and heard, creates safety and space to share one's intimate, guilt-

and shame-ridden thoughts (Siegel, 2010). Applying elements of attachment theory in interplay with systems theory allows for new relational experiences, while also creating a space for developing new meaning and understanding related to previous experiences. It is not a person's previous experiences but the way the person reflects on those experiences that affects parenting (Stern, 2004). This creates reflexivity in the sense that action and thought follow each other in this interplay. Understanding is connected to recognizable and actual actions, which makes it easier to convey what is experienced in each specific interaction situation. This can lead to a reorientation without reluctance to expand the context of relational interaction, which will thus not only involve fear and threats, but also care and safety. It is the parents who must take care of the child, which emphasizes the importance of seeing parallel processes in therapy. It is important to develop the stories and expand the context by co-creating further narratives about who was also present, and is now present, among family members, friends/networks and care providers. Also important is a focus on strengths and possibilities for coping, as well as the identification of relational interaction patterns and attachment processes in the family that are important to carry forward (Dallos & Vetere, 2022). Systems theory will help us to retain the complexity and introduce new understandings. The context will affect the possibility of parents attaching to their children and will also influence how far and in what ways the attachment relationship will impact the children's development (Belsky & Capaldi, 2009). In this way, relationships are established in interaction in a specific context, where it is not just a question of psychological capacity. The hope is that the therapy will create a relational foundation containing elements of safe attachment experiences, which will enable parents to see themselves in the important relationship with their children in a way that promotes development.

A key aspect of this approach is to heighten awareness of how our cultural preferences influence the point of view we choose, which may become the most relevant and important part of the counselling. By exploring our preferences in a self-reflexive way, we can become more aware of what cultural influences and dominant discourses do to us. As a therapist, the most important questions related to "new horizons" that arose for me in talking to Hanne and Martin were: how small is big enough for an intervention, how can I help the parents to become confident enough to share their stories and how to get help to notice their internal working models and a learned parenting style. Similarly, the recognition of the love that lies in daring to accept help and putting one's life in the hands of others was also a topic of conversation (See also chapter on Agape).

By helping Hanne and Martin to talk together, and exploring the various factors involved, I was in a position to challenge discourses and norms and to discuss topics not mentioned. In this way, families can be helped to explore their own challenges without increasing their stigma. These parents know that their lifestyle is viewed negatively in relation to unspoken norms and prevailing discourses about parenthood, and parenthood in combination with substance use. If we as therapists do not see this, there is a risk that the way of life of such families and parents is not explored and understood on their own terms, which means that therapists are unable to help these clients (Aamodt, 2009).

An important aspect of the therapy is to explore how we as professionals relate to the families. We should be aware of the risk of removing parts from the whole, leading to less communication of an overall picture of the situation. This may mean that families adapt and relinquish parental responsibility, while we should be helping them to have the attitude: "we are the parents". By failing to deal with inequality, we risk reaffirming disparities, reinforcing vicious circles and stigma and thus inflicting further shame, stigma and guilt on parents. There is thus a danger of increasing the burdens they already carry (Aamodt, 2009; Gullestad, 1989). One question that the therapist and the parents considered was how to co-create a suitable framework. How can the therapist position herself to enable her to explore what the parents describe? Important perspectives were also greater awareness of what it means to acknowledge one's power as a professional (Aamodt, 2009; Foucault, 1980).

A key theme of the counselling sessions was: *How can we help the parents to adopt the child's perspective?*

Helping Hanne and Martin to feel safe and to recognize and express their own motives was an important perspective in the sessions. Being in a dialogue that acknowledges and appreciates people implies an approach with the belief that it is possible to create change. Bringing hope into the dialogue helped the therapist to focus on building bridges and strengthening the parents' resilience factors. It was vital to create a therapeutic space where the parents could gain new, positive relational experiences. The alternative is that the therapist could be overwhelmed by the complexity, instead of considering how small is big enough. If the therapist and the family co-create the therapeutic situation, new relational experiences can take place.

The therapist said to Hanne and Martin; I really like your way of speaking about your feelings of fighting spirit and your strong wishes to fight for Ina. Let's explore together what that might mean. Here, the therapist is reflecting the parents in a positive sense, which encourages hope and belief in change; the belief that one can become a good enough parent. Faced with complex problems, therapists are often eager to help but run the risk that different interventions disrupt each other. It is important to link up the various fragments of observations and experiences to ensure that the understanding of how small can be big enough is established as a common understanding.

Concluding Remarks

I have used the sessions with Hanne and Martin to show how counselling parents can be understood as a circular process, which can be combined with a social constructionist and systemic approach. The starting point for this chapter was to show what kind of focus can be large enough in sessions with parents with substance use in an inpatient unit for parents and children. The parents are there to receive help to cease their substance use, in addition to help in assessing whether their care and parenting can be good enough. I have shown how an approach based on the systemic paradigm is possible, despite the fact that such treatment units are often a normative context with the power to assess whether the clients' parenting is good enough or not.

Hanne and Martin knew best the kind of life they wanted, and they were experts in their own areas, while the therapist facilitated an open dialogue and process. I have tried to show how therapist and client can co-create a space that allows for the sharing of perspectives, to enable them to find a way forward together. The parents' challenges are illustrated through various statements about what they wanted to get help for, and what they were afraid of in encounters with therapists, child welfare services and treatment facilities. This approach can be a useful contribution and point out new horizons that open up new opportunities in therapeutic work with parents and children. Seeing things as they are, with their limitations and possibilities, engenders hope, the hope of starting a lasting change in the factors that affect parenting. The need to have nuanced understandings of the interaction between parents and children, and between parents and therapists, was thus a key priority in the sessions with Hanne and Martin.

References

Aamodt, I. (2009). Grenser for makt og Ansvar. Institusjonelle ramme-betingelser og praktisk handling i samarbeidet mellom barnevernstjenesten og psykisk helsevern for barn og unge [Limits of power and responsibility. Institutional frameworks and practical action in collaboration between child protection services and child and adolescent mental health services]. (Bup). *Fokus på Familien, 37*(1), 3–18.

Anderson, H. (2003). *Samtale, sprog og terapi. Et postmoderne perspektiv* [*Talk, language and therapy. A post-modern perspective*]. Hans Reitzels Forlag.

Andersen, T. (2005). *Reflekterende prosesser. Samtaler og samtaler om samtalerne* [*Reflective processes. Talk therapy and talk about talk therapy*]. Dansk Psykologisk Forlag A/S.

Andersen, T. (2011). Et samarbeid av noen kalt veiledning [Cooperation, also called guidance]. In M. H. Rønnestad, & S. Reichelt (Red), *Veiledning i psykoterapeutisk arbeid* [*Guidelines for psychotherapeutic work*]. Universitetsforlaget. Kap. 6

Bakhtin, M. M. (1981) *The dialogic imagination* (M. Holquist & C. Emerson, Trans.). University of Texas Press.

Belsky, J. R., & Capaldi, D. M. (2009). The intergenerational transmission of parenting. Introduction to the special section. *Developmental Psychology, 45*, 1201–1204.

Bordin, E. S. (1994). *Theory and research on the therapeutic working alliance; New directions* (A. O. Horvath & L.S. GreenBerg, Eds.).

Bowlby, J. (1998). *A secure base. Parent–child attachment and healthy human development.* Routledge.

Dallos, R., & Vetere, A. (2022). *Systemic therapy and attachment narratives: Applications across a range of clinical settings* (2nd ed.). Routledge.

Felitti, V. J., & Anda, R. F. (2010). The relationship of adverse childhood experiences to adult health, well-being, social function, and healthcare. In R. A. Lanius, E. Vermetten, & C. Pain (Eds.), *The hidden epidemic: The impact of early life trauma on health and disease.* Cambridge University Press.

Foucault, M. (1980). Truth and power. In C. Gordon (ED.), Power/knowledge: Selected interviews and other writings 1972–1977. *The Harvester Press Limited.*

Gergen, K. (2010). *Relationel tilblivelse: videre fra individ og samfund* [*Relational becoming: Moving on from individual and society*]. Dansk Psykologisk Forlag.

Gullestad. M. (1989) *Kultur og hverdagsliv* [*Culture and everyday life*].

Johnsen, A., & Torsteinsson, V. (2012). *Lærebok i familieterapi* [*How to conduct family therapy*]. Universitetsforlaget AS.

Lock, A., & Strong, T. (2014). *Sosialkonstruksjonisme. Teorier og tradisjoner* [*Social constructionism. Theories and traditions*]. Fagbokforlaget.

Myra, S. M., Ravndal, E., Torsteinsson, V. W., & Øfsti, A. K. S. (2018). Pregnant substance abusers in voluntary and coercive treatment in Norway: Therapists' reflections on change processes and attachment experiences. *Journal of Clinical Nursing, 27*, 959–970. https://doi.org/10.1111/jonc.14067

Myra. S. M. (2017). An approach to supervision practice with therapist who work with pregnant substance abusing women in voluntary and compulsory treatment setting (pp. 185–194). In S. Vetere & J. Sheehan (Red), *Supervision of family therapy and systemic practice.* Springer.

Reading, B. (2002). The application of Bowlby's attachment theory to the psychotherapy of the addictions. In M. Weegmann & R. Cohen (Eds.), *The psychodynamics of addiction* (pp. xviii, 178 s.). Whurr.

Siegel, D. J. (2010). Commentary on "Inergrating Interpersonal Neurobiology with Group psychotherapy": Reflections on mind, brain, and relationship in group psychotherapy. *International Journal of Group Psychotherapy, 60*(4).

Stern, D. N. (2004). *The present moment in psychotherapy and everyday life.* Norton & Company.

Søderstrøm, K., & Skårderud, F. (2009). Minding the baby: Mentalization-based treatment in families with parental substance use disorder: Theoretical and conceptual framework. *Nordic Psychology, 61*(3), 47–65. https://doi.org/10.1027/1901-2276.61.3.47

Vetere, A., & Stratton, P. (2016*). Interacting selves. Systemic solutions for personal and professional development in counselling and psychotherapy.* Routledge.

White, M. (1984). Pseudo-encopresis: From avalanche to victory, from vicious to virtuous cycles. *Family System Medicine, 2*(2), 150.

White, M., & Epston, D. (1990). *Narrative means to therapeutic ends.* WW Norton & Company.

Wiig, E. M., Halsa, A., Myra, S. M., & Haugland, B. S. M. (2018). Rescue the child or treat the adult? Understanding among professionals in dual treatment of substance-use disorders and parenting. *Nordic Sudies on Alcohol and Drugs, 35*(3), 179–195.

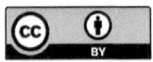

5

Families Living with Anticipatory Grief; How Can We Both Understand and Explain?

Anne Grasaasen

Max and his dad arrived first. It took half a year, and then Martin came along with his mother. It appeared that both boys had a progressive neurological condition stemming from their parents both being bearers of a special gene. A review of their heredity revealed that they were fourth cousins. The process in the period preceding the deaths of the children was extremely demanding. The boys moved gradually backwards developmentally. They lost their vision, language, bodily control and developed dementia. Their parents had been sweethearts from their early teenage years. Despite their great love, they now found themselves toxic for one another. Through a difficult but friendly process, they chose to divorce and to take primary responsibility for one child each. Max and Martin died at 10 and 12 years old respectively.

A. Grasaasen (✉)
Department of Family Therapy and Systemic Practice, Faculty of Social Studies, Oslo, Norway
e-mail: anne.grasaasen@vid.no

© The Author(s) 2024
S. M. Myra et al. (eds.), *New Horizons in Systemic Practice with Children and Families*, Palgrave Texts in Counselling and Psychotherapy, https://doi.org/10.1007/978-3-031-38111-9_5

69

I am concerned with practice, also in terms of how it is related to research. When families are living in such a complex and demanding lifeworld as Max, Martin and their parents, we need to stretch in all directions and search for the best of all that is available to provide help for those who need it. Understanding people in demanding life situations is a work of interpretation that demands both knowledge and experience. More than anywhere else, I feel here the importance of the not-knowing position (Anderson, 1997) in which my role as therapist is as an artist of conversation, and my competence lies in facilitating dialogue. In a situation characterized by dramatic changes in the lifeworld of the family, I must listen actively both to what is said and what is left unsaid. The conversational space must be kept open enough to encompass difficult questions, those for which there might not be any answers. It must encompass causal explanations that *do* provide answers. It must offer sufficient peace for us to search for meaning, and there must be space enough to accommodate strong emotions. Meeting Max, Martin and their parents, as well as other families living in similar lifeworlds, has strongly influenced my clinical and academic work. Clinical experiences have become issues for research and developmental work and then feed back into my practice.

In my role as an artist of conversation with Max, Martin and their parents, I have found particularly helpful social constructionism's focus on the power of dialogue to open up a multiverse. This has allowed me to perceive family-professional exchanges as encompassing both explanation and understanding. In encounters, our shared search for a multiverse appears liberating because it creates a wide-angle perspective. When we become curious instead of critical about how people engage in one another's reality, we open for the assessment of alternative paths (Anderson, 1997). My understanding of the social constructionist perspective gives me courage, acceptance and belief in the power of dialogue.

Illness Phenomena: A Meeting of Medical and Phenomenological Perspectives

Illness as a phenomenon encompasses different dimensions of human life, and as a phenomenon, it consists both of narratives and physiological conditions. A lifeworld such as that which Max, Martin and their parents must manage brings with it a need for knowledge and help with medical, psychological and social arenas. The more intricate and complex the condition, the greater the need for thoroughness in finding ways to provide a holistic service. The challenges faced by the family, therefore, also involve ideas not immediately embraced by systemic perspectives. Families do not need either-or, but both: to explain and to understand. In my effort to keep family-professional dialogues open to the multiverse with families like this one, I have found resources in the work of medical philosopher Fredrik Svenaeus (2011) who views these ideas as well-suited to achieving an understanding of the special requirements of lifeworld's altered by serious illness. Being the parent of a dying child can be experienced in terms of existential threat that becomes anchored in the body as physical pain and despair. The threat of the loss of a child can be experienced as an existential crisis in which *being-in-the-world* changes character and becomes *unhomely* in a threatening and chaotic manner. For parents, explanations are sought in which the *chaos story* can be made more understandable and eventually replaced by a *restitution narrative*. Svenaeus also describes a third type of narrative, the *quest narrative,* the path between these two. In this story, parents can redefine the situation from threat to one in which they can find new meaning because the meaning structure of narrative can be opened, unpacked and displayed in new ways (Svenaeus, 2011).

> *Mother*: What was so strange was that they didn't find anything wrong, not on the tests, not in the pictures. And then of course you think, there's nothing wrong, it'll probably be fine. But then everything got worse. When the boys finally got the diagnosis, we screamed non-stop for two days. I remember the feeling of waking up but still being caught in the nightmare. It was as though someone ripped the rug out from under my feet, and underneath there wasn't a floor, just a black hole.

Therapist: Yes, that must have been terrible to find out. You got the worst answer you could get to your questions. I think what you experienced is every parent's worst nightmare, only it was really happening, and there was nothing you could do. When you think back, what made you nevertheless begin to move up out of that black hole?

Mother: It was hard, because I kind of couldn't see any meaning in doing it. But, at one point I was completely exhausted by being in so much pain, and I realized it couldn't get any worse. That was a turning point in fact. I had gotten the answer I feared the most, but getting an answer was still easier than feeling the fear of getting the same answer.

Therapist: Yes, sometimes we really must go to the uttermost limit no matter how painful it is. What made you able to think differently despite such great pain?

Mother: I read about anticipatory grief, and then I thought, yes, that's exactly how I feel. There are others who understand, who know how I feel. That helped me to understand why I reacted as I did. I also read about other families and found comfort and help in what they said. But I also felt guilty, then, about my boys. While I'd been more concerned about death than living, they needed me more than ever. It was about more than just me. I began to think more about what I could do so that they could feel as good as possible.

Diagnoses are descriptions and categorizations of symptoms, and they function in part to legitimize treatment and the need for types of help (also see the chapter from Axberg and Petitt in this volume). With a basis in natural scientific research and experience, statements can be made about how a condition will develop, the possibilities for treatment interventions and prognosis. In encounters with people and illness states, there is therefore a logical breech in the statement that diagnoses are not realities. As systemic therapists, we must acknowledge that they also represent ways of being in the world and describe perspectives existing in and important to the lifeworlds of many people. At the same time, I will always challenge categorizations that over-simplify people or situations, or in which the explanations provided appear limited to cause and treatment, with lifeworld and context relegated to the background. Descriptions of people will always stand in relation to something greater, to the relation between us, to discourses and to the context that frames the situation. As therapists, we must therefore ask ourselves questions about whether these constructions are helpful and related to what the family is seeking help with, or answers to. Max and Martin's mother felt particularly helpless in the search for a diagnosis and reached a turning point when this frustrating process could finally be concluded. She was told that there was no cure and that her children's lives would be short. Hope disappeared, forcing them to construct new boundaries around a lifeworld in which death had become the frame for life. This medical approach, nevertheless, contributed important answers.

It is important to emphasize the special features of diseases in which hope of improvement is absent and diminishing or loss of function is a part of disease development. When death is the frame of life, conversations always have a context in which drama is present to a greater or lesser extent. In parallel with advanced medical treatment, there is a continuous need for help in creating new constructions of how to live, and the creation of meaning will be a dimension of continual significance (Grasaasen, 2020). By expanding the description of the disease with images that embrace a greater unity of the lifeworld, a more caring encounter can be constructed. Michael White (2008) describes traumatic events such as being thrown into a fast-flowing river after which the only thing one can manage is to hold one's head above water. To get the ground under one's feet, one must climb up onto the riverbank. It is only when one can stand safely that it is possible to find the adequate emotional distance to be able to speak about these experiences and achieve meaningful understanding of what has happened. According to Jerome Bruner (2003), it is then our narrative gift that can give us the strength to accord meaning to experience. Lived life is expressed through narratives in which events are pieced together into meaningful stories. When a breech or a turning point occurs, this structure brings a useful means of embracing complex experiences and renders them understandable. After the impact of the diagnosis, the mother climbed up onto the riverbank to firm ground, from which point meaning construction resulted in the development of a coherent story that, no matter how tragic, could make family life worth living. As their therapist, it became important at this point to maintain the dialogical space and meet this private tsunami with conversations that acknowledged reality. In subsequent conversations, we slowly changed focus from support and comfort to searching for words that, with incremental steps, produced movement and hope for change in the direction of a new way to live everyday life. We highlighted resources both in the mother herself and in the environment that could make daily life manageable. Attention to living in the now helped her identify meaningful experiences to share as a family that simultaneously created memories for future recollection.

Therapist: When you talk about how you got through this early time, I think that you must have found enormous power from somewhere. What is this strength of yours, do you think?

Mother: I don't know, and it's not every day it works, either. It doesn't take much before I'm standing on the edge of the hole again. I really just want to carry the boys around in my pockets all the time, because I know that they won't get to be adults. I can still get completely overwhelmed with desperation about the fact that they're going to die. But I think there is a strength in knowing I'm the one who can make their lives as good as possible. And that there's nothing else I'd rather use my energies for than doing just that. I want them to have the best, and that means they need me.

Therapist: So, your days are unstable, and some days are more difficult than others. At the same time, I think that I hear that you have great awareness of your own feelings and reactions. What makes it possible for you to keep far enough away from the edge that the grief feels manageable?

Mother: It might sound strange, but I'm glad that we didn't lose the boys in an accident or something like that. I think it would've been harder. I'm grateful that I have the chance to prepare myself for losing them. Now time feels a little borrowed. I don't want to waste it. It has taken on a unique value that I guard.

Therapist: So, being able to prepare yourself for the fact that they will die helps you to live in a way? To value each day?

Mother: Yes. I wake up of course always with restlessness in my body, but then I force that away and begin to think about what might be fun to do that day. It doesn't have to be so much, but I try to create precious moments every day. I feel the best those days I manage to do this. Knowing that time is limited helps me to take care of them.

Therapist: So, you look for valuable moments that both make the day a good one and that you can take with you further. Can you describe a moment like that?

Mother: Yes. We always get up early in the morning because that's when the boys are in the best shape. Today, we sat around the breakfast table even though they only get fed through a tube in their stomachs. I lit candles with a match and then I pretended that it was them who blew it out. Then they got to smell that strange smell. Small things like that.

Therapist: That was a small, beautiful story about the small things. Max and Martin are lucky to have such help to fill their days with sensory, meaningful experiences.

Mother: I'm not always so active though. Some weekends when we haven't done so much, I'm really pleased just because we've felt good.

A social constructionist, relational approach to grief and death free people from the clutches of individualistic, pathologized versions of grief that insist on a final stage of acceptance. In conversations with parents, I have been inspired by Lorraine Hedgke (2021) and what she calls re-membering conversations. Instead of the adage that *the human being is born and dies alone*, Hedtke locates narrative relational perspectives of life as those that are foundational; all of us are born into an interconnected web of other people. Stories about relationships are resources that strengthen and highlight life as a circular narrative, without beginning or end. In re-membering conversations, narrative conversational practice is used to create active stories about a fellowship that continues after death. Questions that build bridges between the past and the future have the aim of creating narratives that can continue to include the dead child in the lifeworld of the family. The conversations can give strength and power to the parents by calling forth *memories of belonging* instead of *creating distance* to a loved child. Knowing that they are allowed to *not forget* can be the source of peace. Parents can find a way to go on with the dead child *beside them* instead of having to *put it behind them*. Children can continue to warm their parents' hearts by actively being included in meaningful stories and as part of the lived life of the family (Hedgke, 2014).

Emotions—And the Curse of Dualism

Mother: You hold your hands in front of you like a bowl and try to carry water. Regardless of how hard you hold, it always drips through a little bit. So, with each drop, and it's Max and Martin I'm holding, a little more of them drips through every single day. It happens so slowly that it takes a while before I notice they've lost more function, and when I register that now they can't do what they could yesterday, or last week, I get so sad.

There's a saying that grief is the price of love and the cost of being lucky enough to love. In that perspective, grief is part of life as a normal and appropriate adaptive process to life without the loved one. The narratives of parents in anticipatory grief are often saturated with metaphors. They speak about *moving through unknown territory* in a *journey without a map, filled with unpredictability* towards a death they know will occur. They feel fear and desperation, so much so that they *do not have energy* and *feel drained* (Grasaasen, 2020). Feelings are abstract, and the use of metaphors is an effort to grasp the ungraspable through using more concrete references in a transformation that makes them understandable. Love and grief are not psychological entities hidden in consciousness, but rather ways to behave that are visible on the outside of the person (Grasaasen, 2022). At the same time, existential thoughts about life and death arise, as well as a continuous stream of new questions about how to cope with life.

Even though the methods of natural science have shown their value in describing genetic and biological processes, this value can be correspondingly poor when describing challenges at the psychological and interpersonal levels. Through the monological or "thing-language" of science, explanatory models have been proposed in which phenomena such as anticipatory grief and love have been defined, diagnosed and explained in terms of numbers and categories. Discourses about grief have been directed traditionally towards the experience of loss, pain and longing. With the help of modernist metaphors, we are told we must *let go, get over it* and *move on* (Hedgke, 2021). Harlene Anderson (1997) calls this pathologizing language, or the "language of inadequacy", one that is usually static and looks for causes with little room for understanding. Anderson uses a similar metaphor to that used by Max and Martin's mother when she points out that such language has a psychological effect that can best be depicted as a *black hole*, from which there is no liberation or possibility of meaningful action. I have never heard parents say that they either can or will let go of the loved child. That they will *get over it* has no meaning for parents or for me as a therapist. On the contrary, I have learned that each unique lifeworld provides unique life-knowledge. I have found that maintaining an attachment to the living is more protective than *letting go*. It can make a difference when we find a way to speak about our children that can carry memories of them on in the lives of parents as part of the story of the family about itself.

Therapist: I am impressed about how you reflect around – and manage - your days. At the same time, I think that you can do this because you're so strict about what you allow yourself to think about and do. I think this might get very demanding over time, and that it will be easy to strain yourself. You give so much to others and need to get something back. You also need acknowledgement for what you do. Who is there for you? Who sees what you do and fills up your storehouse with energy when you need it?

Mother: Even though we're separated, I can share almost everything with my boys' father. He's a very good dad to them and a co-parent with me. We share love for them and grief over losing them. And then I have my mother.

Therapist: In what way is she there for you?

Mother: She says that I'm the best mother in the world. She tells me all the time how proud she is of everything I do for Max and Martin. She puts up with all my bad days and I never need to feel guilty when I complain to her. She's super important to me.

Therapist: So, your mother is someone you can always lean on when you need to. I'm glad to hear that. I also think that Max and Martin would say exactly the same thing about you. Are there other people who are significant, and who you know are there for you?

Mother: It always does me a lot of good being with these others who have children with the same diagnosis. The other parents. Our children are completely different just like other children are completely different. We parents are very different from one another too. We are a good, broad demographic group with completely different interests, and completely different backgrounds. But we have a common bond that is very strong. Being with other people who are going through the exact same thing as you are, is very healing. It's essential for coping with life, actually.

A dimension of therapeutic significance is the facilitation of conversations with other parents in similar situations. Such fellowship represents a special form of experiential knowledge in which language becomes a shared feature and the experience of living in anticipatory grief is subsequently recognizable without requiring many words or explanations. Heidegger (Lock & Strong, 2010) calls language *the house of being* in which we reside through social interactions and as response to our participation in life. Narratives of others can resonate and become understandable because they represent lived life that can communicate unspoken knowledge (Grasaasen, 2020). Even though parents are continuously overwhelmed by their emotions, the situation can change from one of *threat* to one of development of understanding in which *being-in-the-world* takes on a new shape (Svenaeus, 2011).

The Power of Language and the Force of Dialogue

To speak is silver; to listen, gold. Each is both a challenge and an important part of the art of conversation. How we use language is thus essential to the creation of good conversations. Language is descriptive but also functional as linguistic action, because implicit to its use is used in a particular context. We use it to perform actions such as to inform, explain or comfort. Thus, words are never neutral, and they have distinct consequences.

Mother: I'm grateful to be able to talk with you too. You know, after we were told about the boys' diagnosis, no one else has talked with us about death. You are the only one who mentions the word. When I'm at the hospital, my feelings are stirred up and I cry a lot. I feel that the people who work there feel that's difficult. I think maybe they avoid talking about things that make me show my feelings.

Therapist: I'm glad that our conversations are experienced as good, but I'm not sure I'm equally satisfied about why. Instead of getting help from those who should be there for you, you find you need to take care of them?

Mother: Yes, it feels that way. Sad stories, no one likes that. We all would rather hear that things go well in the end. It's hard of course in this situation.

Therapist: That is very sad that you have to go through that. No matter what it might concern, this isn't a burden you should have to carry.

Mother: No, but I have so many questions, there's so much I wonder about that even you can't help me to get answers to. It's not what I want, but now and then doubts about how the future will be push their way in. The boys have become heavier to manage and don't have as much space in our laps as before. It's as though their lives only just fit into a child's body. I wonder about how their lives will end, how that will happen. I think it's scary and frightening to think about. It's those sorts of things I could have used someone to ask about.

In meetings with parents, verbalization of relational experiences occurs, and reality is understood through speech acts. The way we speak will influence how the situation is experienced (Alvesson & Sköldberg, 2018). This aspect is particularly important in connection with disease and death. Parents in anticipatory grief seldom have the energy to be attentive to language and slide easily and unnoticed into whatever linguistic universe is offered to them. As conversation partners, we have both power and responsibility—"Words can bewitch us", warns Wittgenstein (1969). Escaping the word-games in which we participate is just as impossible as moving pieces in a chess game any way we wish. We allow ourselves to be seduced into following the rules without thinking that we can simply just reject the whole game. The relational focus in dialogue and in social construction affords acceptance of a multiverse of meanings. When Sheila McNamee (2004) uses the term promiscuous to challenge us to cooperation this is so that we can be open to other theories as discursive alternatives. Cooperative constructions can improve our ability to be relationally engaged with those we are to help. We become sensitive to their stories as well as to our own in ways that allow us to be both receptive and relationally responsible (McNamee & Gergen, 1998). In encounters with difficult life situations, it is therefore a strength to question one's own ideas and remain open to the possibility of having different conversations. When we attempt to develop meanings that can be helpful to parents, it is their narratives that must be the conversational axis and their reality that is acknowledged (Anderson, 1997). It is interesting for me to note a sort of circular connection in this between the complexity of anticipatory grief and my own experience as therapist. Elements from different theoretical positions become complementary rather than contradictory, and multiple phenomena are then available for reflection. As a therapist, I can relate to the disciplinary perspectives I find useful instead of working on behalf of a single position. Max and Martin's diagnosis can be understood both as socially constructed and brought into existence by basic structures. In meetings with their parents, I can understand anticipatory grief as a biological basic structure that is part of what it means to be human, but which finds expression in relation to the social constructions of which the person is part. This is a matter both of nature and culture, explaining and understanding.

The narratives in the text are fictional composites using elements drawn from different conversations with several parents. I have learnt so much from these, and I am very grateful for them Thank you to everyone!

References

Alvesson, M., & Sköldberg, K. (2018). *Reflexive methodology: New vistas for qualitative research.* Sage.

Anderson, H. (1997). *Conversation, language and possibilities: A postmodern approach to therapy.* Basic Books.

Bruner, J. (2003). *Making stories: Law, literature, life.* Harvard University Press.

Grasaasen, A. (2020). How to live on borrowed time? A parent perspective on anticipatory grief. *Fokus på familien* (pp. 96–114). Universitetsforlaget.

Grasaasen, A. (2022). My mother, my mirror? Three generations encounter family therapy. *Journal of Family Therapy, 44*(4), 462–473. https://doi.org/10.1111/1467-6427.12413

Hedgke, L. (2014). Creating stories of hope: A narrative approach to illness, death and grief. *Australian and New Zealand Journal of Family Therapy, 35*, 4–19. https://doi.org/10.1002/anzf.1040

Hedgke, L. (2021). From a individualist to a relational model of grief. (S. McNamee, M. Gergen, C. Camargo-Borges, & E. F. Rasera, red.). *The Sage handbook of social constructionist practice*. Sage.

Lock, A., & Strong, T. (2010). *Social constructionism: Sources and stirrings in theory and practice*. Cambridge University Press.

McNamee, S. (2004). Promiscuity in the practice of family therapy. *Journal of Family Therapy, 26*, 224–244.

McNamee, S., & Gergen, K. J. (1998). *Relational responsibility: Resources for sustainable dialogue*. Sage.

Svenaeus, F. (2011). Illness as unhomelike being-in-the-world: Heidegger and the phenomenology of medicine. *Med Health Care and Philos, 14*, 333–343. https://doi.org/10.1007/s11019-010-9301-0

White, M. (2008). *Traumer, narrative behandling av traumatiserte opplevelser [Trauma, narrative treatment of traumatized experiences]* (D. Denborough, Red). Dansk psykologisk Forlag.

Wittgenstein, L. (1969). *On certainty*. Blackwell Publishers.

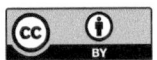

6

Tailoring Treatment in the Context of a Manual: A New Horizon for Family Therapy with Families with a Young Person Suffering from an Eating Disorder

Vigdis Wie Torsteinsson and Gina Hægland

Introduction

Aurora, 15 years old, lives with her father and mother in an apartment in a big city. Aurora has an older brother living at home and an older sister living in another city. The parents have only recently understood that Aurora has a restrictive eating problem. Both feel guilty for not having seen what was happening earlier. The mother tells us that she suffered from an eating disorder herself some years ago, and that her experience with the health care system was rather poor. This experience has made it particularly difficult for her to trust the therapist's credibility in helping Aurora. Her own knowledge and experience with healing from an eating disorder play an important role in the therapeutic process. Aurora shows limited self-awareness of being sick. Her BMI (Body Mass Index) is, by the time she was referred, 15,8.

V. W. Torsteinsson (✉) · G. Hægland
BUPA, Sykehuset i Vestfold, Tønsberg, Norway
e-mail: psykologspesialist.haegland@gmail.com

© The Author(s) 2024
S. M. Myra et al. (eds.), *New Horizons in Systemic Practice with Children and Families*, Palgrave Texts in Counselling and Psychotherapy,
https://doi.org/10.1007/978-3-031-38111-9_6

The gap between science and clinical practice has somehow got lost in the debate about evidence-based practice and the use of manuals. Clinicians know that, even though we are fairly faithful to the manual's guidelines, we are still experiencing difficulties in adaption to the needs of individual families. The knowledge covered in a manual is just one of many competencies we are using in our meetings with families and clients (Fruggeri, 2012; Fruggeri et al., 2022). We need a new perspective, a new horizon to handle the dilemmas between established empirical knowledge and the adaptions to the specific needs of the individual family. This chapter introduces a tool that may be useful in this important, but challenging task. We are using the Family-Based Treatment manual (FBT) and the work with eating disorders as an example. The work described is nevertheless applicable to other contexts of trouble and other manuals as well.

The treatment with the highest level of empirical support for adolescents below 18 years with a short duration of illness is Family-Based Treatment (FBT; Couturier et al., 2013). Our first meeting with Aurora and her parents followed the interventions underscored in the FBT manual. We underscored the seriousness of the situation, instructed the parents to take responsibility for Aurora's meals and meal plans and gave them information about the importance of underweight reduction for recovery. The manual will be described in greater detail later.

But this way of working did not work well with this family. They returned some days later, the parents desperate and angry with each other. Aurora had shut down and would not say much. The parents told us that they found it difficult to do things in a way that made Aurora comply with their instructions. Instead, their meals had ended in tears and anger and had not resulted in an increase in Aurora's diet. They partly blamed the strict criteria of the manuals' interventions. Mother even cited the title of an article she had found on the Internet: "This must be somebody else's roadmap" (Conti et al., 2017)!

This is a common concern amongst therapists working within the frames of a manual. To some families, the instructions seem to worsen what they already experience as difficult and traumatic. Even if the FBT-interventions are efficient (Couturier et al., 2013), still only about 50% of the families involved have success. The authors of the manual conclude like this: "We do know that efficacy data for FBT, especially adolescent AN, are quite robust, even though remission rates remain elusive for more than half of all cases. While preliminary, moderators of FBT for adolescent AN have been identified and could aid us in determining the most (or least) responsive patient groups… What we do not know, yet, is whether specific adaptations to manualized FBT will confer improved remission rates" (Lock & Le Grange, 2018). The modifications we have seen so far are mostly additions given as an extended therapeutic period, e.g. CBT, RO-DBT, etc. Some of these are added because of an uncertainty about whether the FBT takes good enough care of the youth's needs.

Our intention with this chapter is to create some ideas about a new horizon in working within the framework of a manual. The FBT manual works as an example, but the points we underscore can be useful in any manualized context. We will suggest a possible way to modify the manual without removing the efficient factors that have been the core of the positive FBT results. That means focusing on what we so far know about the success factors, combined with ideas that can be positive modifiers of the stringent manual in order to individualize interventions to each family and arguing for these modifications as possibilities to make family therapy an even more efficient intervention for the families who need our assistance. And we will get back to Aurora and her family later.

Eating Disorders

First: a short introduction to eating disorders. They are dangerous illnesses with potentially high mortality rates, potentially long-term medical consequences and a high risk for chronification even for adolescents. Early and adequate interventions reduce these risks. In recent years, we have seen an intensified effort to find effective interventions to help families who are affected. The illness has a great impact on the whole family, both on parents (Rhind et al., 2016) and siblings (Fjermestad et al., 2020).

As with many problems that affect young persons, eating disorders put parents in a position of helplessness and despair. The overwhelming anxiety parents may experience reduces their ability to take efficient action against the illness. When parents doubt their own strength or skills to counter the eating disorder, the fear of making the situation even worse also follows. This uncertainty gets stronger due to changes in the young person. Parents often describe this as a big change in personality: from an independent, caring, responsible position to a bewildered young person with one goal in life: to reduce the intake of food as much as possible.

From the young person's perspective, the reduction in food intake often goes together with what they believe is a solution to something they perceive as a problem. Lack of self-confidence, wanting more friends, being more attractive or more able to "deliver" on various social media platforms or in activities related to sports amongst a lot of other possible perspectives—perspectives that are important to a young person who is striving to feel good enough to live a satisfying life. Citing Sarah: "it doesn't help if my mother tells me that I am good enough! Of course she would say that – she is my mother, that's what mothers do!!!" It is the judgement of her peers that she wants to influence. And it is a perspective that most young persons will recognize as an important goal. The problem arises when this goal overshadows everything else in life, including the big health hazards. And that is when we would say that the young person is overtaken by the eating disorder, not able to recognize any other perspective on his or her life. Even when life itself is reduced to avoid eating, and every other aspect of life is ignored, including school performance, friends and family, or being able to participate in activities that up to this point have been a source of enjoyment, the eating disorder is not recognized as an enemy.

The Manual

FBT is an outpatient treatment which utilizes the adolescent's family as a resource in re-feeding and recovery (Lock & Le Grange, 2013). The earliest studies of family therapy for anorexia nervosa were conducted at the Maudsley Hospital in London. This approach was subsequently adjusted somewhat, given a more behavioural focus, and called FBT at

Stanford University and The University of Chicago in the United States (Rienecke & LeGrange, 2022).

Therapy is conducted in phases. The first phase focuses on achieving weight gain through giving parents responsibility for the young person's eating and meal-related behaviour. In the second phase, responsibility is gradually returned to the young person (Lock & Le Grange, 2013). Phase three focuses on developmental themes such as independence, social behaviour or sexuality (Lock & Le Grange, 2013). The actual developmental issues addressed depend upon the needs of each family (Medway et al., 2019).

The FBT manual has elements from several family therapy approaches and is based on 5 fundamental assumptions:

1. the therapist holds an agnostic view of the cause of the illness;
2. the therapist takes a non-authoritarian stance in treatment;
3. parents are empowered to bring about the recovery of their child;
4. the eating disorder is separated from the patient and externalized; and.
5. FBT utilizes a pragmatic approach to treatment, with the focus on the here and now (Rienecke & Le Grange, 2022).

Several of these assumptions have been shown to be related to the success of FBT, e.g. agnosticism (Lock et al., 2020), externalization (Lock et al., 2020) and parental competence (Robinson et al., 2012).

The five fundamental assumptions show how FBT represents a combination of elements from several family therapy traditions. First, the basis is structural family therapy, where the hierarchy in the family is underscored, and the parental system has a different kind of responsibility than the children. The strategies designed to give parents increased agency related to the eating disorder are linked to this tradition. Parental confidence regarding how to handle meals and food intake is an important success factor. Aurora's parents were instructed to take responsibility for her meals to secure a sufficient nutritional intake. Included in these instructions is the therapist's conviction that they have the necessary strength and willpower to do this. The agnostic and pragmatic approach to the problem and the therapeutic process reminds us of solution-focused therapy, insisting on the futility of understanding the causes of the eating disorder, and that therapy must be concentrated on what are useful steps to reduce the influence of the eating disordered on the young person and the family. The therapist's non-authoritarian and consultative stance reminds us of the systemic and the dialogic-collaborative approach to the therapeutic process which views the family's own resources and responses as the key factors securing therapeutic success.

One of the changes that was introduced in the manual developed in the United States, was a stronger focus on behavioural change. This is particularly evident in Phase 1, with, as we have seen, the concentration on giving the parents confidence in their ability to take control of the young persons' meals and food intake and securing a weight gain in the young person. The reason for this is of course that early weight gain is an important predictor of outcome (Doyle et al., 2009; Le Grange et al., 2014). At the same time, many of the families who have not experienced FBT as useful emphasize that a one-sided focus on weight gain has not given them the therapeutic platform they needed in their efforts to combat the eating disorder (Conti et al., 2017). So, is it possible to expand the focus in the start-up phase so that both therapist and family can navigate within a new horizon, a larger room for action than the manual recommends?

The Active Elements in FBT

Some of the active elements in the FBT manual are, as we have underscored, the importance of parents being the driving force in the reduction of the eating disorders influence, the active focus on reduction of underweight, and the change of behavioural patterns related to the reduction of eating. This did not work for Aurora's family and still is insufficient for a large number of families.

So how can this situation be improved? Is it possible to see a new horizon where a greater percentage of the families troubled by eating disorders can be helped? The following is a summary of a large Norwegian study of families that have been through several treatment processes at different levels of service:

...former inpatients prefer tailored treatment and a collaborative approach. Eight subthemes constituting two main themes emerged: *1) There are no ready-made solutions. Staff should facilitate collaboration by tailoring treatment toward the young person's perspectives, and 2) Emphasizing skills that matter. Staff should display a non-judgmental stance, educate patients, stimulate motivation, enable activities and prevent iatrogenic effects during the stay.* (Nilsen et al., 2019)

The young persons also underscore a real dilemma that is clinically easily recognizable. They want and need the support and determination of their parents/family, but they also "place a distinctive emphasis on self-responsibility and determination" (Nilsen et al., 2020). This has been a point of interest for years although little has been done to secure the young person's active contributions with their perspective as part of the process in the early phases (Krauter & Lock, 2004).

The Challenges of Using a Manual

Based on group data, a manual gives the therapist a structure and an overview that has been documented as useful for many families. But group data are often not a sufficient basis for interventions in the individual family, even if they have been useful for a large percentage of the families that have been involved in the actual studies. To clinicians, who want to be useful to as many families as possible, there often has to be room to adjust and to take into consideration the specific needs and wishes of the individual family. To achieve this, it must be possible to take into account the specific therapeutic context that the therapist team and family develop together and to the special needs that the individual family presents (Robertson & Thornton, 2021).

The relationship between following the manual from step to step and the outcome of therapy is complex. There is a multitude of factors that can influence the relationship. Included in these factors are the kind of therapy that is offered, the concrete problems that each family brings with them to therapy, the alliance between the family and the therapists, and the young person's motivation to help create change. If the young person is negative to any kind of change, being true to the manual can be counterproductive, or, at best be an ineffective strategy. The young person with an eating disorder is often identified with the eating disorder and sees the eating disorder as their own project associated with some aspects of their lives that they want to improve. Even if the parents most of the time are very motivated to create changes in a very troubling and scary situation, the young person's engagement in the healing process is important for long-term changes to occur (Nilsen et al., 2020). In Aurora's family, a number of these points could be the reasons for them not having the intended effect of the manual's directions.

In the therapeutic context, we would like to turn the attention from following the manual letter by letter to a process that is more flexible and tailored, but which nevertheless takes into account the active ingredients in the manual that are documented by the empirical research. How can we connect and create a dialogue with Aurora and her family in a way that helps us to be useful to them? In addition, we think that this approach to a greater degree underscores the importance of the therapeutic alliance (Robertson & Thornton, 2021). The increased attention to the young person's perspective also makes it possible to focus to a greater extent on their motivation for change (Nilsen et al., 2019).

Another argument for being flexible and individualizing treatment is presented by Medway et al. (2019). The aim of their study was to let parents and young persons describe the different ways that AN impacts adolescent development, and how FBT helps families out of the eating disorder. The informants describe three distinct ways, relating to different meaning context in the young persons and the families' lives (called developmental difficulties by the authors). "For some young people, FBT plays a key role in easing their return to activities that promote healthy development, or in adjusting their relationship with their family of origin to be more developmentally appropriate. For others, the role of FBT is largely limited to weight gain; however, this can allow young people to find their own path back to healthy development post-treatment" (Medway et al., 2019). In this way, the meaning context associated with the eating disorder onset can give valuable (and necessary) clues as to what changes the family needs to work on to get rid of the ED.

Suggestions About How to Customize the Manual to Meet Individual Families Needs

So how can we base our treatment on the strong involvement of the parents, together with a collaborative stance where the young person also is invited to participate, and help them take a stance against the destructive forces of the eating disorder together? From our perspective, working with a systemic formulation at the start of treatment could be a way to open possibilities to expand and go beyond the manual without neglecting the active and efficient ingredients of the manual. It gives us the possibility to work with the will (and wish) to cooperate in the family, which is a success factor in any family therapy process (Friedlander et al., 2011). In addition, it includes the young person's voice in an early part of the process to a much greater degree.

A systemic formulation is, from this stance, a therapeutic tool that can help the therapist bridge the gap between the manuals' more generic guidelines and the here and now unique meeting with the family (Baudinet et al., 2021). We have chosen to work with a systemic formulation to underline both the theoretic baseline, the context in which it is made and the way it is carried out. We need something more to help us navigate in the uniqueness and complexity that each young person and family represents. We need something that can translate the general guidelines into appropriate idiosyncratic judgements about what to do.

Manuals are designed to ensure that families and clients are given evidence-based help for their presented problems. Despite this, the tool the manual is given through is inevitably the therapist (Blow et al., 2007). This influences the way the manual and the therapy are provided in the real world. As therapists, we use clinical judgements based on more than the manual at hand. We are, amongst other things, driven by well-rehearsed habits, personal preferences and other blind spots. A systemic formulation ensures that the therapists' ideas are openly shared. The family are given the opportunity to contribute to the dialogue with additional and relevant information and to be active participants in the process. The systemic formulation ensures that we involve the family as active participants and collaborators.

So, what exactly is a systemic formulation? A systemic formulation can, in a broad sense, be described as the process in which the therapist, together with the family, tries to make sense of the situation (Baudinet et al., 2021). We, as well as the family and the young person are, by virtue of being human, always searching for meaning. A systemic formulation is a way to formalize this natural search for how things are connected. Through this collaborative exploration, the aim is to end up with a current plan helping the young person get well. This plan is based on general knowledge about eating disorders, the FBT manuals active ingredients, and the information from the family and the young person that has evolved through the formulation process. The process was initially inspired by Baudinet et al. (2021) and is further developed from other written sources on formulations (Johnstone & Dallos, 2014; Kennerley et al., 2016) and adapted to our local clinical culture and practice.

The formulation work we have adopted has naturally evolved into two separate phases. The first phase is an exploring conversation structured around some core features. The first step in this phase is to create a genogram. The genogram is made to get an overview of the young person's family and network. In the following steps, the genogram will function as a stepping stone into the different categories of interest. Circular questions facilitate an exploring conversation.

The conversation covers some core elements that are integrated in the systemic formulation, but does not necessarily follow a strict, sequential order. The aim is to create a common understanding between the therapist and the family. The best way to manage this is to follow the family in their preferred directions. At the same time, the therapist takes responsibility for covering the structure inherent in the systemic formulation. The conversation is predominantly fueled by circular questions to bring forth the family's reflections, experiences and assumptions. For example, how does it make sense that the young person has developed this particular eating disorder, what and who affects the current problem, what made the eating disorder develop in the first place and what makes it so hard to escape from it? It is important to emphasize that the purpose here is to ask for the family's *understandings*. Not to find "the real causes" for the disease. This is an essential part of all systemic practice and in agreement with the agnostic attitude of FBT.

When the genogram is drawn, the next step is to explore the family's experience of the current difficulty (Baudinet et al., 2021; Kennerley et al., 2016). This will, in our context, normally present itself as different stories of troublesome eating behaviours or distorted thoughts connected to food and body image. We have found it useful to adapt the four steps in Michael Whites externalizing map in this part of the formulation (White, 2007). That is, first, collaboratively find a proper name for the problem; second, explore the effects it has on the young person and the important relationships in his or her life. Third, ask the young person to evaluate the effects and, finally, ask for a justification of this evaluation to bring forth the young person's values, dreams and preferred ways of living. This part of the systemic formulation supports the FBT manual's emphasis on using an externalizing language and lays the foundation to maintain an externalizing language throughout the whole therapy process. It also helps the therapist and the parents to discover any possible motivation the young person may have for getting well. During the exploring conversation (the first part of the systemic formulation) the following themes should also be covered to get as rich a picture as possible; triggers, modifiers, precipitants, vulnerability factors, protective factors and perpetuating patterns (see Fig. 6.1).

Based on the length and focus of this chapter, we choose to limit ourselves to describe how the systemic formulation can influence how we work with the effects of the perpetuating patterns and can have relevance for facilitating and adapting a unique treatment process.

The perpetuating patterns are in line with circular hypothesis and with FBT agnostic stance and pragmatic approach to treatment. They can give the therapist and the family a way to collaborate to explore what keeps the problem going, and to discover what natural interventions these patterns invite us to do, to break the vicious circles. In other words, they are important in making concrete plans. The perpetuating patterns we create together with the family should reflect the information given throughout previous conversations. Some perpetuating patterns recur in most eating disorders. This applies, for example, to the pattern created by being in a biological state of starvation (see Fig. 6.2). These patterns are part of the FBT manual and must be presented by the therapist as important knowledge. Other patterns are unique to the individual

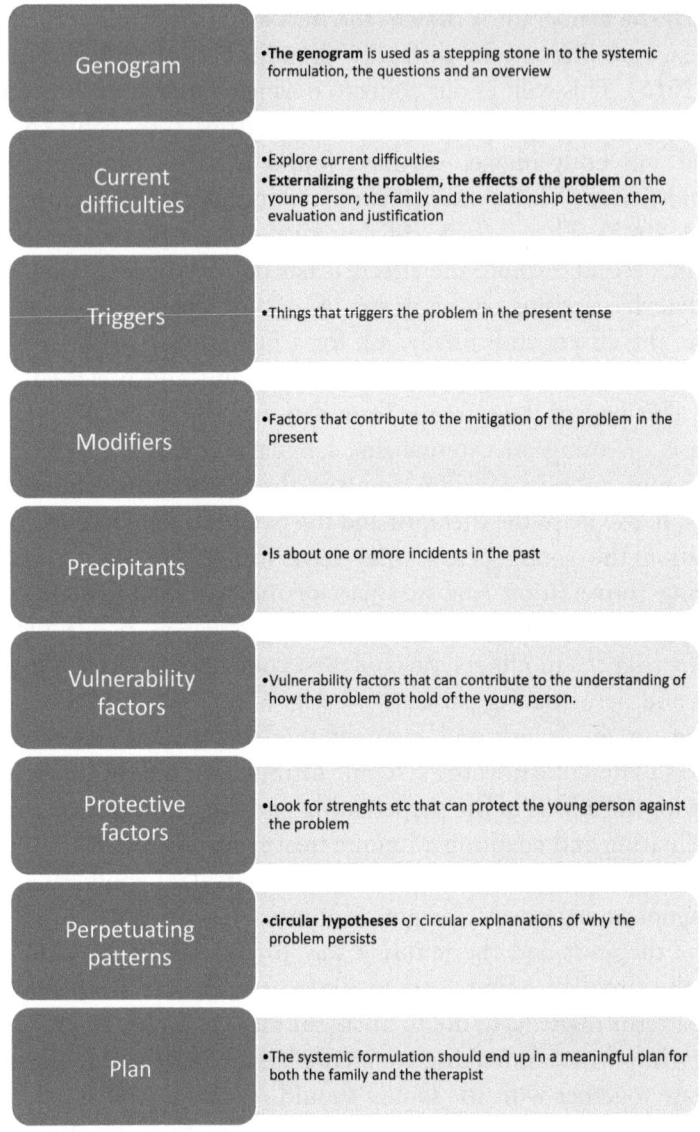

Fig. 6.1 A template formulation 1

young person or family and are more to be discovered. The clinical case described below will show an example of this.

The second phase of the systemic formulation is to create a visual picture of the information given in the first phase (see Fig. 6.3). This can be done in different ways. Our example is just one way to provide a pictorial synthesis of the information. The purpose of this phase is to collect the most important information available at that time in collaboration with the young person and his or her family to make a tailored plan. This plan is the result of a cocreation of meaning during phase 1 and should make sense to the family and be in line with what they believe in. It is made through a coordination of meaning and knowledge from the family and the therapist.

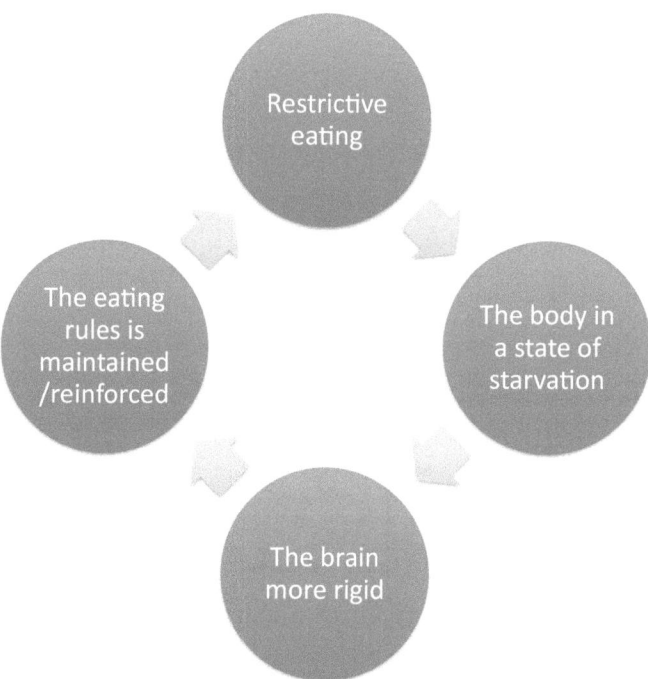

Fig. 6.2 An example of a perpetuating pattern

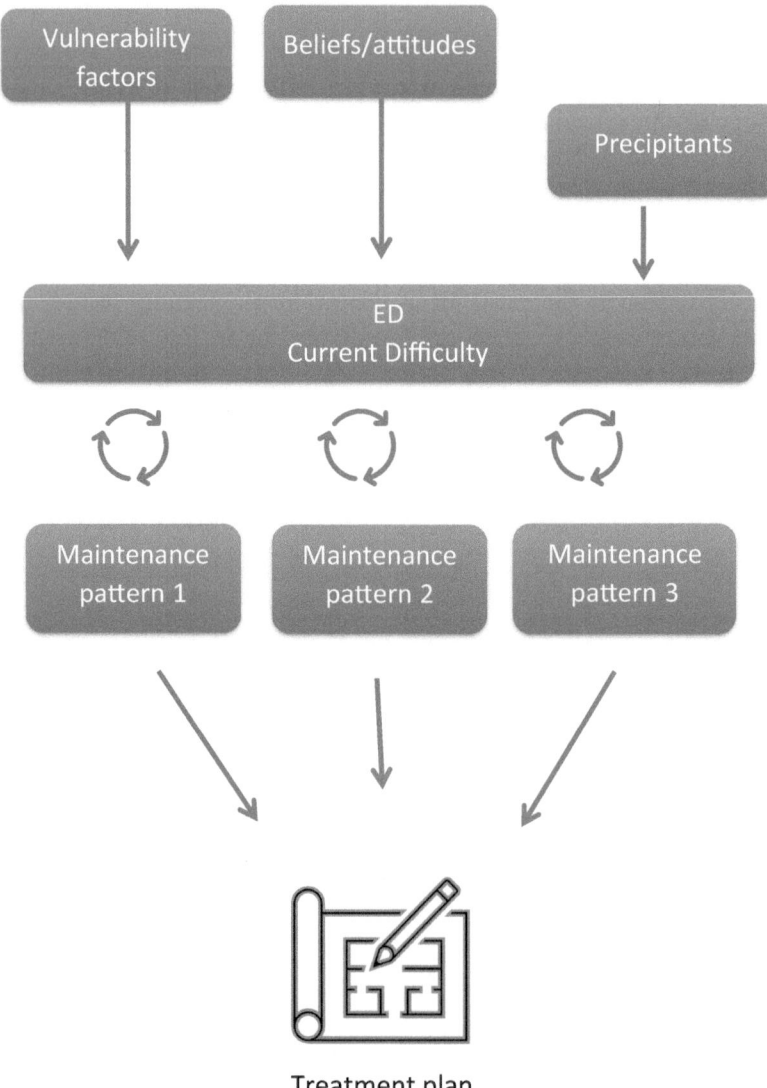

Treatment plan

Fig. 6.3 A template formulation 2 (inspired by Kennerley et al. 2016)

An Example of a Systemic Formulation Process

But let us return to Aurora and her family, restart the therapeutic process and give both therapists and family a new horizon for their cooperation. In the new first session with the family, we drew a genogram. One important vulnerability factor that emerges during this session is Aurora's bad experiences with peers during her early school years. She has several experiences of being shut out and exploited by supposedly close friends. The parents show grief for all the pain she has suffered. Despite these experiences, Aurora described herself as quite extrovert. She has just started high school when we meet them. Some of her friends from secondary school have left the city to study in other parts of the country. Aurora is ambivalent regarding this. She misses her friends, despite the difficulties that have been, but is, according to herself, also looking forward to a fresh start with new friends. Her parents express great concern regarding drop out and lack of social belonging if the eating disorder makes it difficult to attend school. In a way, it seems even more important to the parents that she attend school than Aurora. Aurora is explicit about her wish to manage school but is also clear about the costs. The manual instructs the therapist to advise reducing school attendance until the weight reduction is stopped and reversed. The parents think that school attendance is crucial for Aurora. Aurora is ambivalent. Is this challenge part of the reason why therapist and family are not moving forward?

Therapist: So, tell me, Aurora. How did all this start? Do you remember?

Aurora: I don't really know. But I think it was like a solution for me. I didn't know how to fit in. I felt different and didn't know how to connect to the others and eating less and getting thinner was a way to cope, I guess. I tried to get thinner to make them see me...

Therapist: So how did the Solution help you? Did It help you in relation to your peers?

Aurora: No, I guess not, but it made me feel better...

Therapist: In what way?

Aurora: I guess it made me less vulnerable. I coped, and I wasn't dependent on the others in the same way as before. I felt stronger...

Therapist: What can I call this Solution, Aurora? Is it ok by you that I call it an eating disorder?

Aurora: It is more like an eating challenge

Therapist: Ok. So, this eating challenge, does it help you or does it make it more difficult for you to get to know your new peers?

Aurora: I don't know. It feels difficult to be me. My head goes blank, and I am afraid they think I am stupid...

Mother: That's because your energy level is low. It will be better as soon as you gain some weight. You will be fine...

Therapist: So, how does this feeling of going blank affect the eating challenge? Does it make you want to eat more or less? Or none of them?

Father: She has never eaten a lot, actually...

Therapist: (to father) So, does that mean that you think the feeling of blankness is not connected with the eating challenge?

Aurora: You don't understand (to father). It does makes it more difficult to eat!

Therapist: And how does that effect the interaction with the others?

Aurora: What do you mean?

Therapist: Does it make you feel stronger and safer in the interaction with the others? Like at the onset of the eating challenge. You said that on the onset it made you feel stronger. Is it the same now? Or is it different? Does it, in some way or another, affect the feeling of being disconnected from them?

Aurora: I really want to get to know then, but I don't feel like me. I feel sort of numb and disconnected and feel stupid. But I don't want to give up. I really want to belong to the group, just like they do...

Therapist: It sounds like the eating challenge disturbs your wish to connect to your new classmates. Is that so?

Aurora: Maybe. But I am not sure it is all about the eating challenge...

One dilemma that occurs during the initial formulating conversation was whether Aurora should attend school at this stage of her illness or not. Given Aurora's low BMI, and her low food intake, our normal advice would be to limit school attendance. But given the information about her earlier history, her explicit wish to connect with peers and the parents' conviction about the importance of her going to school, made us hesitate. This was reinforced by the mothers own bad experiences with the health care system, her personal competency regarding eating disorders and her reluctance to give us authority. This was an example of a discrepancy between the manual's guidelines and the family's unique history and its implications. The following dialogue shows how the exploration of some of the perpetuating patterns gave us an opening to establishing an agreed upon plan for the following weeks.

> *Therapist*: To me it sounds like we are talking about two different self-perpetuating patterns. One good and one less good. The good pattern captures a wish that you have been explicit about (to parents). Because of Aurora's painful history from previous school years, it makes it important for you to give her the opportunity to have a good start in this new school. By letting her attend school as normal, you hope to give her the opportunity to establish new friendships, that hopefully promotes a better life for her in general, improves her self- esteem and hopefully makes it easier for her to eat.
>
> *Father*: Yes, that's right…
>
> *Therapist*: (to Aurora). What do you think Aurora? Does it feel important to you, as well?
>
> *Aurora*: I guess so…
>
> *Therapist*: So, this is one possible, and wished for development for all of you. On the other hand, you (Aurora) have said something about the struggle you are exposed to attending school these days. And that leads me to the other possible, but more vicious perpetuating pattern. May I say something about that one as well?
>
> *Mother*: Of course…
>
> *Therapist*: Even though the hoped-for consequence of attending school is to help Aurora to get well, it might also be that her current energy level is too low to allow this to happen. It might be that, as she says, she struggles too much to be present in a way that helps her. It might be too tiring for her, and it might drive her into a vicious circle where all her energy goes to a project that doesn't succeed, that makes her feel as a failure amongst her peers and makes it even harder to eat. It might trigger her original solution to eat less to have control in an overwhelming and difficult situation, which sabotages the sufficient weight gain, and might prolong the time she stays sick. How can we make sure to be wise in our next step? The margins aren't too good, so we have to make sure we don't try something that doesn't work for too long. What do you think?

Mother: I think that we must see a weight gain in one or two weeks, that she has a better mood, and that she manages to eat without too much trouble

Therapist: That sounds like a feasible plan? You (parents) let Aurora have the chance to get into the positive effects of attending school, by letting her attend full time for one or two weeks. If Aurora continues to show negative signs on those three parameters, then we must reconsider the plan? Is that so?

Therapist: (to Aurora): How does this plan affect you? Can you do this? And how can mom and dad notice or even help you if the struggle gets too tough before next week?

Aurora: Now that I think they understand that this is not all about the eating challenges, I want to try, and I wish they will let me do it. I think they will notice if the plan doesn't work, and I think we all want to give it a try!

The parents agreed on giving the plan a try for the two weeks. They came back for a new appointment the next week. Aurora had gained 700 grams, and the parents thought her mood had become better. Aurora hadn't noticed any difference, but she was still determined to try another week. We met weekly for a long period and followed up the three parameters every session. Aurora gradually gained weight, and the conversations turned in other directions. We made another systemic formulation at this point. Our experience was that we had a good and safe working alliance with both Aurora and her parents. The themes that Aurora brought forth were painful and demanding for all to talk about, but they were an important part of her healing process. Our experience was that the formulations helped us make the context, the dialogue and the collaboration good enough to help Aurora get well in a rather smooth way.

Concluding Comments

Our intentions with this chapter have been to show how a modification of the original FBT manual can help us develop our treatment processes in a way that makes the resources of both the family and the therapist team important ingredients in planning and implementing a constructive dialogue and the feeling of cooperation. That is, to create a new and wider horizon to ensure cooperation and dialogue as the decisive element in establishing a foundation for a working alliance for the family.

The FBT manual underscoring the importance of a consultative stance encourages a cooperative stance from the therapist team. Through our examples, we hope to show that a less instructive stance than the manual prescribes can be beneficial to the process, and still make room for the knowledge and experience in the therapist team. We hope this can be the start of making the FBT manual a useful intervention for a larger group of families that struggles with restrictive eating disorders in a young person. We also hope that it can inspire therapists working with other manuals to expand their work in similar ways.

References

Baudinet, J., Simic, M., & Eisler, I. (2021). Formulation in eating disorders focused family therapy: Why, when and how? *Journal of Eating Disorders, 9*, 97. https://doi.org/10.1186/s40337-021-00451-3

Blow, A. J., Sprenkle, D. H., & Davis, S. D. (2007). Is who delivers the treatment more important than the treatment itself? The role of the therapist in common factors. *Journal of Marital and Family Therapy, 33*(3), 298–317. https://doi.org/10.1111/j.1467-6427.2007.00375.x

Conti, J., Calder, J., Cibralic, S., Rhodes, P., Meade, T., & Hewson, D. (2017). 'Somebody else's roadmap': Lived experience of Maudsley and family-based therapy for adolescent anorexia nervosa. *Australian and New Zealand Journal of Family Therapy, 38*(3), 405–429. https://doi.org/10.1002/anzf.1229

Couturier, J., Kimber, M., & Szatmari, P. (2013). Efficacy of family-based treatment for adolescents with eating disorders: A systematic review and meta-analysis. *International Journal of Eating Disorders, 46*(1), 3–11. https://doi.org/10.1002/eat.22042

Dallos, R., & Stedmon, J. (2014). Systemic formulation: Mapping the family dance. In L. Johnstone & R. Dallos (Eds.), *Formulation in psychology and psychotherapy: Making sense of people's problems* (2nd ed.). Routledge.

Doyle, P. M., Le Grange, D., Loeb, K., & Doyle, A. C. (2009). Early response to family-based treatment for adolescent anorexia nervosa. *International Journal of Eating Disorders, 43*(7), 659–662. https://doi.org/10.1002/eat.20764

Fjermestad, K. W., Rø, A. E., Espeland, K. E., Halvorsen, M. S., & Halvorsen, I. M. (2020). "Do I exist in this world, really, or is it just her?" Youths' perspectives of living with a sibling with anorexia nervosa. *Eating Disorders, 28*(1), 80–95. https://doi.org/10.1080/10640266.2019.1573046

Friedlander, M. L., Escudero, V., Heatherington, L., & Diamond, G. M. (2011). Alliance in couple and family therapy. *Psychotherapy, 48*(1), 25–33. https://doi.org/10.1037/a0022060

Fruggeri, L. (2012). Different levels of psychotherapeutic competence. *Journal of Family Therapy, 34*(1), 91–105. https://doi.org/10.1111/j.1467-6427.2011.00564.x

Fruggeri, L, Balestra, F., & Venturelli, E. (2022). *Psychotherapeutic competencies: Techniques, relationships, and epistemology in systemic practice.* Taylor & Francis.

Johnstone, L., & Dallos, R. (2014). Introduction to formulation. In L. Johnstone & R. Dallos (Eds.), *Formulation in psychology and psychotherapy: Making sense of people's problems* (2nd ed.). Routledge.

Kennerley, H., Kirk, J., & Westbrook, D. (2016). *An introduction to cognitive behavior therapy: Skills and applications.* Sage.

Krauter, T., & Lock, J. (2004). Is manualized family-based treatment for adolescent anorexia nervosa acceptable to patients? Patient satisfaction at the end of treatment. *Journal of Family Therapy, 26*, 1. https://doi.org/10.1111/j.1467-6427.2004.00267.x

Le Grange, D., Accurso, E. C., Lock, J., Agras, S., & Bryson, S. W. (2014). Early weight gain predicts outcome in two treatments for adolescent anorexia nervosa. *International Journal of Eating Disorders, 47*(2), 124–129. https://doi.org/10.1002/eat.22221

Lock, J., & Le Grange, D. (2013). *Treatment manual for anorexia nervosa: A family-based approach* (2nd ed.). The Guilford Press.

Lock, J., & Le Grange, D. (2018). Family-based treatment: Where are we and where should we be going to improve recovery in child and adolescent eating disorders. *International Journal of Eating Disorders, 52*(3), 481–487. https://doi.org/10.1002/eat.22980

Lock, J., Le Grange, D., Accurso, E. C., Welch, H., Mondal, S., & Agras, W. S. (2020). Is online training in family-based treatment for anorexia nervosa feasible and can it improve fidelity to key components affecting outcome? *Journal of Behavioral and Cognitive Theraphy, 30*, 75–82.

Medway, M., Rhodes, P., Dawson, L., Miskovic-Wheatley, J., Wallis, A., & Madden, S. (2019). Adolescent development in family-based treatment for anorexia nervosa: Patients' and parents' narratives. *Clinical Child Psychology and Psychiatry, 24*(1), 129–143. https://doi.org/10.1177/135910451879 2293

Minuchin, S., & Fishman, H. C. (1985). *Family therapy techniques*. Harvard University Press.

Nilsen, J. V., Hage, T. W., & Rø, Ø. (2019). Minding the adolescent in family-based inpatient treatment for anorexia nervosa: A qualitative study of former inpatients' views on treatment collaboration and staff behaviors. *BMC Psychol, 7*, 72. https://doi.org/10.1186/s40359-019-0348-2

Nilsen, J.-V., Hage, T. W., Rø, Ø., & Halvorsen, I. (2020). External support and personal agency—Young persons' reports on recovery after family-based inpatient treatment for anorexia nervosa: A qualitative descriptive study. *Journal of Eating Disorders, 8*, 18. https://doi.org/10.1186/s40337-020-002 93-5

Rhind, C., Salerno, L., Hibbs, R., Micali, N., Schmidt, U., Gowers, S., Macdonald, P., Goddard, E., Todd, G., Tchanturia, K., Lo Coco, G., & Treasure, J. (2016). The objective and subjective caregiving burden and caregiving behaviours of parents of adolescents with anorexia nervosa. *European Eating Disorders Review*. https://doi.org/10.1002/erv.2442

Rienecke, R. D., & Le Grange, D. (2022). The five tenants of family-based treatment for adolescent eating disorders. *Journal of Eating Disorders*. https://doi.org/10.1186/s40337-022-00585-y

Robertson, A., & Thornton, C. (2021). Challenging rigidity in anorexia (treatment, training and supervision): Questioning manual adherence in the face of complexity. *Journal of Eating Disorders, 9*, 104. https://doi.org/10.1186/s40337-021-00460-2

Robinson, A. L., Strahan, E., Girz, L., Wilson, A., & Boachie, A. (2012). 'I know I can help you': Parental self-efficacy predicts adolescent outcomes in family-based therapy for eating disorders. *European Eating Disorders Review, 21*, 108–114. https://doi.org/10.1002/erv.2180

White, M. K. (2007). *Maps of narrative practice*. Norton. https://doi.org/10.1176/ps.2008.59.8.941

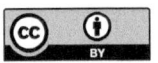

7

Systemic Perspectives and Psychiatric Diagnosis: Mutually Exclusive or Mutually Inclusive?

Ulf Axberg and Bill Petitt

Summary

In the discussion below, we argue for the position that a system of diagnostic categories is necessary for all psychotherapists, in a parallel but different manner to the way in which it is important for medical practitioners. We systemic therapists also have a fundamental need of organizing the domain of human suffering so that we can bring order to

U. Axberg (✉)
Department of Family Therapy and Systemic Practice, Faculty of Social Studies, VID Specialized University, Oslo, Norway
e-mail: ulf.axberg@vid.no

B. Petitt
Logos AB, Lerdala, Sweden
e-mail: bill.petitt@telia.com

© The Author(s) 2024
S. M. Myra et al. (eds.), *New Horizons in Systemic Practice with Children and Families*, Palgrave Texts in Counselling and Psychotherapy,
https://doi.org/10.1007/978-3-031-38111-9_7

our clinical practice, our research and our professional communication. The most important question is "how?"

Throughout this chapter, the reader should bear in mind that we discuss this issue primarily as systemic psychotherapist in considering how we may think of the ICD/DSM categories—we offer no critical analysis of how other professions think of or use them, but focus only on their relevance for the practice of systemic psychotherapy. It is also central to our systemic perspective that any attempt to understand human emotional suffering, based on only one perspective such as biology, psychology or sociology, will necessarily be incomplete. One practical example of what acceptance of such a presupposition would suggest is that no single domain of knowledge that studies human beings can claim the sole right to interpret and control the meaning of any diagnostic system of categories for everyone. It is rather up to members in each domain to decide the nature of its relationship to the categories and to arrive at their own considerations concerning meaning and value. This also applies of course to specialist sub-domains—such as those found under the class of psychotherapies: no single model or approach can claim universal precedence and retain credibility. It perhaps is as Onnis (2016) suggests, that what we have learned so far from the study of complex and dynamic systems teaches us that a plurality of perspectives is necessary to understand them. The eventual value of any single perspective will perhaps have to be valued in other terms—for example utilitarian ones (Jablensky, 2016; Kendler, 2022).

Introduction

In common with most others who work in the field of mental health, we (the authors of this chapter) have been obliged to develop a professional relationship with the two dominant diagnostic guides in use today— the International Classification of Disease 10 (ICD-10: World Health Organization, 1992, 1993) and the Diagnostic and Statistical Manual of Mental Disorders 5 (DSM-5: American Psychiatric Association, 2013). Several of the chapters in the present volumes describes working as systemic therapists in relation to mental health as well as other diagnosis, see for instance the chapters by Grasaasen and Benestad Pirelli, Grasaasen, Myra, Wie Torsteinsson and Hægland, de Flon and Sheehan. We are both psychotherapists, with a professional perspective that is anchored in family and couples (systemic) therapy. While we concur with the widely held view that there are many problematic issues connected to both diagnostic systems, many of the conflicts generated within the mental health field that we are aware of seem to emerge from the different meanings that are attributed to them and/or the ways in which they are applied. One obvious example is that many people seem to think that the diagnostic categories to be found in the manuals identify and describe illnesses—something that the authors themselves explicitly say that is not what they do. Interestingly, the word "diagnosis" stems from two Greek words *dia-* (through, thoroughly) and *gignoskein* (to know, perceive). Thus, its central meaning could be conceptualized as "to learn about the nature of a phenomenon thoroughly". As stated above, our major focus in this chapter is on the diagnostic systems themselves and how we might think about them, not on how they are used in different contexts.

It is of interest to note that the diagnostic categories described in ICD and DSM in one sense reflect our everyday need for specific words or names for identifying different kinds and classes of experience (or different kinds and classes of anything). The giving of names provides a kind of verbal shorthand when anchored in shared culture that we use in our personal narratives when describing the experience of self and others: "I feel depressed", "She is autistic". In folk psychology—the non-expert, public narratives used to describe and explain experience—their general acceptance is probable evidence that they possess an important functional value. This means that a systemic therapist, even when working in settings other than a strictly psychiatric one, will often encounter language-usage that identifies different forms of diagnostic categorization. In clinical practice, we cannot escape this—so we need a strategy to accommodate it into our daily work.

DSM and ICD are the dominant diagnostic guides created and published by the American Psychiatric Association (APA) and the

World Health Organisation (WHO) respectively. While DSM exclusively presents categories concerning mental disorders, ICD-10 (and its successor, 11, which is not yet universally applied) also includes most known diseases. Chapter 5 in ICD is devoted to "Mental, behavioral and neurodevelopmental disorders", which approximates the same area of study as DSM (when we use the name ICD in the present text, we are referring only to Chapter 5 unless otherwise stated). For the purposes of this chapter, we shall consider the two sufficiently similar in content that they can be discussed as if they are—or as the authors of DSM-5 put it, "… the salient differences between the DSM and the ICD classifications do not reflect real scientific differences, but rather represent historical by-products of independent committee processes" (American Psychiatric Association, 2013, p. 11). Together the two manuals are central to the field of mental health, a position often strengthened by law as well as by their application to establish and justify political planning, resource sharing, organizational routines, research, diagnosis and treatment, epidemiological studies and professional communication. It is, in fact, difficult to imagine a world without their ubiquitous presence. Despite this, there are possibly few established manuals that attract so much debate and criticism.

This chapter will describe some of the ways in which we (the authors) have learned to relate to and live with DSM/ICD. To do so, the principal perspective we employ is that of the philosophy of science, which encourages us to think about how we think—a meta-perspective familiar not only to philosophers, but also to systemic psychotherapists. As both DSM and ICD represent formal attempts to categorize a specific part of the natural world, we begin with a general discussion about the nature and function of categories.

The Nature and Function of Categories

Day in and day out, our senses are consciously and unconsciously stimulated by a vast number of experiences, while a steady stream of thoughts pass through our minds. We must learn to navigate in a complex world in which danger is an ever-present possibility. One of the most powerful intellectual tools that we possess to help us organize our experience of the world is that of making categories—of sorting phenomena into different groups, where all the selected members of any given group are placed there because they are judged to share specific characteristics or elements which separate them in some distinctive way from other phenomena. We continually employ categories, often without being aware that we are doing so. For example, a mushroom picker has hopefully learned that there is something called mushrooms and that some kinds may be eaten and even that some taste better than others—while knowing that being able to distinguish between edible and poisonous species is as important today as it was for our ancestors.

The creation of a primary category called mushrooms, along with its sub-categories, is one example of knowledge that has been accumulated and organized over time. While the function of the category is obvious, its ultimate value is to be found in how well it serves the needs of both the ones who created it, as well as any others who choose to use it. Categories themselves are usually considered intellectual and social constructs that are used in the process of cognition as it acts on experience, helping to bring some form of order to the latter (Cohen & Lefebvre, 2005; Harnad, 2005; Lakoff, 1987). They influence how we feel, think, behave and relate—and are even used to order the physical world, for example, in the form of standardization (Bowker & Star, 2000). In the case of ICD/DSM, they represent an attempt to organize information obtained from individuals who have sought professional help with their emotional suffering and loss of function. ICD/DSM are therefore basically an attempt to answer the question, "Are there recognizable, recurring patterns to be found in human suffering?"

If we wish to understand why any given system of categories is as it is, and accepting that they are intellectual and social constructs created in a particular social context by someone (or in the case of diagnostic categories, a "group of someones"), for a specific purpose, then we can begin by asking four questions: (1) Who created the system, and in what context? (2) What kinds of things are included/excluded? (3) What is the defined purpose of the system? (4) What are the consequences of its implementation—how well do they match the intended purpose?

1. Who created the system and in what context?

A brief examination reveals that both systems are clearly medically oriented. A look at those who were responsible for and contributed to the latest edition of DSM reveals the following: overall 72% were members of the medical profession and when we examine the composition of The Task Force (those who selected and suggested the contributors) 82% were medical doctors. This composition can only be interpreted and understood as signifying that the dominant paradigm that controlled the creation of DSM-5 was a medical one.

From a gender perspective, it is noteworthy that the DSM Task Force was composed of almost 90% men. Furthermore, of all those who were responsible for and contributed to DSM, 72% were men.

The first of our questions is therefore simply answered: DSM was created by (mostly) male medical doctors. It is free for everyone to imagine what might have been the case if the categorization had been carried out, for example, by female philosophers! (The list of principle investigators at the end of ICD is comprised of 100% doctors, with gender unknown as they are identified only by initials before their surnames.)

Some Reflections

Couple and Family therapy (CFT) was widely criticized in the 1980s and 1990s for, amongst other things, failing to consider the ways in which gender influences roles and relationships (Goodrich et al., 1998; Walters et al., 1988 for a contemporary perspective, see: Almeida & Tubbs, 2020; McGeorge et al., 2020). Today, the theory of intersectionality is generally accepted to be an important contribution that helps in understanding the dynamics of both individual and family life in particular, and of society in general. One defining aspect of CFT is to be found in an awareness of the politics of power, both at a macro- and micro-level, embedded in the general framework of human relationships.

Knowing that the diagnostic systems are the brainchildren of a powerful profession that appointed its own members to create them should make us properly sensitive to the possibility that it may contain bias that inclines it towards the best interests of that profession, and possibly towards men as well. Such a bias is found frequently when research examines in the practice of medicine from a gender perspective (Medical News Today, June 2021, October 2021). It is also obvious that we psychotherapists will use the system—when we do—in a somewhat different manner, and for a different purpose, when compared to medical practitioners. There are overlaps, of course: medical doctors may suggest psychotherapy, while psychotherapists may suggest medication. The diagnostic systems are simply created lists: they only possess value—positive or negative—when applied in the real world.

It is worthwhile to note that even within the medical establishment there are both questions and critical opinions concerning current nosologies (lists that categorize diseases). For example, "...diseases (and disorders) are not self-subsisting entities like electrons, gold and species. They are processes existing in hosts. Within the larger category of pathological states, such as broken bones and dehydration, many different things are grouped into the subclass called disease. So many different kinds of things are called diseases that few scholars consider the category of disease to be a natural kind...The only viable candidates for natural kinds of disease are individual disease types, such as tuberculosis (an infectious disease) and Huntington's chorea (a genetic disease)" (Zachar & Kendler, 2017, p. 57). History reveals to us that creating and then applying categories to living things and therefore attempting to sort them into types (think of contemporary discussions concerning gender or race, for example), is a very difficult, perhaps even an impossible, task. But at the same time, cognizing requires that we do. Knowing that even within systemic therapy we must use some categorization to help bring order to our knowledge, the challenge is to decide if ICD/DSM can be of value for our work, and if not, what system of categories we propose to use instead (see, for example: Raskin, 2018).

2. What kinds of things are included/excluded?

When we look for definitions of what a mental disorder is in the two manuals, in ICD we are informed that, "These descriptions and guidelines carry no theoretical implications, and they do not pretend to be comprehensive statements about the current state of knowledge of the disorders. They are simply verbal descriptions of symptoms and comments that have been agreed, by a large number of advisors and consultants in many different countries, to be a reasonable basis for defining the limits of categories in the classification of mental disorders" (World Health Organization, 1992, p. 2). It goes on to state: "The term "disorder" is used throughout the classification, so as to avoid even greater problems inherent in the use of terms such as "disease" and "illness". "Disorder" is not an exact term, but it is used here to imply the existence of a clinically recognizable set of symptoms or behaviour (sic) associated in most cases with distress and with interference with personal functions" (ibid., p. 5).

DSM reflects in a similar manner over its own list of disorders, which we can summarize in four points:

I. they seldom have any identified, underlying pathological processes "Until incontrovertible etiological or pathophysiological mechanisms are identified to fully validate specific disorders or disorder spectra, the most important standard for the DSM-5 disorder criteria will be their clinical utility for the assessment of clinical course or treatment response of individuals grouped by a given set of diagnostic criteria" (American Psychiatric Association, 2013, p. 20).
II. they are descriptive categories that seek to capture how the disorder is expressed
III. they represent the best currently available system of categorization and will almost certainly need to be corrected in the future
IV. many specific symptoms are to be found in different kinds of disorder, and "…the boundaries between disorders are more porous than originally perceived." (American Psychiatric Association, 2013, p. 6) (See also: Caspi et al., 2020; Plana-Ripoli et al., 2019)

The original data from which the categories in both manuals are formed has two main sources: reports by patients/clients of their own experience, and/or information about them from significant others—psychosocial data, rather than medical. Simply put, the goal of both systems of categorization is to organize the psychosocial data that medical and other health practitioners have gathered in the course of their work, in a manner similar to the collection and organization of data to be found in all other branches of knowledge. In other words, it is an attempt to bring order to a specific area of human experience using experts predominantly selected from a single discipline.

The authors of both manuals point out the atheoretical nature of their data. The primary category (mental disorders) is the name of the class or set within which different types of psychosocial phenomena are grouped and named (schizophrenia etc.). This means that—once created—neither the primary category nor any of the sub-categories are to be thought of as being necessarily attached to any single domain of knowledge, or to any specific theory. In practice, the diagnosis, once established, can be approached from many perspectives. However, somewhat confusingly, while the authors refer to their categories as being atheoretical, they are referred to as being "nosologies". By definition, nosologies are lists of diseases—so what are neutral, non-theoretical categories doing in a nosology? DSM goes as far as to say, "DSM is a medical classification of disorders" (American Psychiatric Association, 2013, p. 10). This mixing of conceptualization occurs several times, creating confusion in the text's basic contextual marking ("what are we talking about, exactly?") and one possible explanation is that they are the consequences of the medical perspective or bias that the creators of the systems share. At first sight, the methodology used to create ICD/DSM is clear: in the real world, psychosocial suffering and related loss of function have been identified using psychosocial judgements and then grouped into disorders. However, even the use of the term "disorder" is in itself easily made problematic in this context. Wakefield's (1992) words highlight one such issue: "...a disorder is a harmful dysfunction, wherein harmful is a value term based on social norms, and dysfunction is a scientific term referring to the failure of a mental mechanism to perform a natural function for which it was designed by evolution".

This is not hair-splitting. Definitions are important in this discussion, as logically, if we are looking for specific kinds of phenomena to add to our primary category, then we must know what we are looking for, and be provided with a clear description for how to recognize them.

Any proposed category is by definition not a natural phenomenon to be found in the world but is a cognitive construction created by using some form of a priori concept or knowledge (logical or reasoned) or some form of a posteriori knowledge (experiential, empirical). For example, if I wish to categorize clocks, then I must know beforehand what a clock is, what it might look like and perhaps even how it works. In DSM/ICD, the primary category "mental disorder" is identified through two elements: loss of function and distress. The sub-categories are simply refinements of the primary category, trying to group the different ways in which patterns of dysfunction and suffering typically occur. Each category or sub-category is a collection of descriptions of thoughts, feelings and behaviour and nothing more. Discussions concerning causality, nature or aetiology may add to our understanding, and even influence treatment, but are not part of the category itself.

Some Reflections

Knowing from the start how those who created the diagnostic systems describe their reasons for doing so and knowing how they built them, allows us to approach the system on its own merits, in the sense that was intended (For example: Is it logically coherent? Does it fit with existing knowledge? Does it fit with our own experience?). It also helps us to understand if the system as it was originally envisaged is influenced in some way when used in different contexts in the real world. That an idea or an artefact is influenced by who use it is hardly surprising. But in the case of ICD/DSM, what is surprising are some of the claims made by different groups about the nature and purpose of the system itself. Thus, some suggest it is an attempt to "biologize" human experience in general, and human suffering in particular. Others claim it seeks to redefine human pain and loss of function as forms of sickness. No such claims are to be found anywhere in the contextualizing preamble to the texts (Interestingly, no one appears to claim it is an attempt to "psychosocialize" human suffering!).

The two systems of categories are revealed as being both more profound and more trivial if one takes the time to read about the methodology and the amount of work that was put into accumulating the data they contain and then organizing them. The system is, in one real sense, the final product of an enormous amount of qualitative research (as opposed to quantitative research), in which individual stories of suffering and lack of function are first collected and then sorted into recurring patterns, and finally the patterns are named. The end product provides us with a vocabulary that can then be used in our work. We can say to the patient, "You are not alone in your suffering: it belongs to a known pattern that we call X".

We can in this manner, gain strength and clarity in our professional role from the texts themselves. If, for example, the patient asks if depression is a sickness, we can respond by saying that there is no evidence for or against the idea that their suffering is the product of biological pathology. However, identifying the symptoms provided by the patient as a "fit" with the category "depressed" opens up the possibility of a variety of treatments, some medical, others psychosocial. In contemporary Western society, these are the two main perspectives for understanding and treating debilitating suffering; however, the diagnostic systems themselves offer no clue for deciding which perspective is the "right" one—rather there appears to be an appreciation that both should be kept in mind in choice of treatment.

At the beginning of the diagnostic process are personal descriptions of experience provided by the client. On the other hand, we have a long list of categories that the clients experience can be matched against. If a match is made, then we have access to a great deal of knowledge readily available that can (hopefully) help us in understanding the patient's narrative and making decisions about possible treatment choices. In medicine, sometimes a diagnosis suggests a known pathological condition. This is *never* the case for the diagnostic categories contained in DSM/ICD (This position is clearly and simply described in Fiske, 2019; Hickey, 2021). People do not "have" their diagnoses: their experienced symptoms have simply been matched with a specific category. In other words, establishing a diagnosis does not identify the existence of a new phenomenon or specific pathology—ADHD, for example, is only the name of a category, not the identification of some "thing" inside the patient (Hyman, 2010; Kendler, 2022; Werkhoven,

2021). Being matched with a category does not identify specific causes for the experiences shared by the client, it simply offers a shorthand way of naming and identifying their general nature. It is only in the information provided by the patient that we can actually gain some understanding of what it is like to be that person.

3. What is the defined purpose of the system?

Both DSM and ICD are clear about their purpose—they see themselves as providing the foundation for consensual diagnoses: "Reliable diagnoses are essential for guiding treatment recommendations, identifying prevalence rates for mental health service planning, identifying patient groups for clinical and basic research, and documenting important public health information such as morbidity and mortality rates" (American Psychiatric Association, 2013, p. 5). This is the important statistical aspect of both systems: descriptions of experience provided by individual patients will suggest to the physician one of the major sub-categories (such as "Anxiety Disorders" or "Neurodevelopmental Disorders") and then facilitate the identification and naming (diagnosis) of a specific disorder (such as "Selective Mutism" or "Attention-Deficit/Hyperactivity Disorder"). Such a system clearly facilitates the collection and organization of data.

The information generated by using the classification systems can be used to inform us, for example, of the rate (percentage of the total population) of a specific symptom (e.g. depression), its general aetiology, its course, and the success/failure of specific treatments, mortality rates and so on. It is also self-evident that clear categories are necessary for research. Further, the information provided by using the systems is important for governments and other public health planners in making decisions concerning, for example, the allocation of resources. These are not trivial purposes.

As noted earlier, the concept and activity of "diagnosing" consists of trying to match symptom descriptions offered by the client or patient to the descriptions found in the classification systems. This is not always easy. One of the problems, generally accepted, is that the categories themselves are rather unprecise: the two major issues are (a) that the boundaries that should help separate the categories often fail to do so, and (b) the same identifying symptoms are often found in many categories (Allsopp et al., 2019). Some of this lack of precision is presumably an unavoidable consequence generated both by the nature of the data (self-referential, descriptions of subjective experience coded into language by individuals from different cultures, social classes, age-groups, genders and so on) and the subsequent efforts (again using language) of professional healers and researchers to categorize those descriptions. Just as interoceptive sensitivity differs from person to person, so does the meaning derived from it. It is also notoriously difficult to be precise concerning behavioural descriptions. Another more radical criticism suggests that the underlying assumption that behaviour, thoughts and feelings can be thought of to exist in the form of units or blocks is not sustainable.

Both systems use a form of redundancy as one attempt to compensate for this lack of precision. The individual syndromes in each major category contain too much information, and directions are included in the introduction to each separate syndrome which specify how to use this over-abundance. In other words, there are clear rules which must be satisfied before a match can be said to have been found. Once found, the match is then said to constitute a diagnosis.

There are two other major difficulties that can present a challenge to diagnosis. The first is that it is difficult to draw clear boundaries between the specific disorders contained in the sub-categories—in the real world, they tend to overlap with and glide into each other. The second is that it is common for patients to present "mixed" descriptions, meaning that their ongoing experience can fit with two or even more categories. When this is the case, it is referred to as comorbidity or co-occurring disorders—and indeed would seem to be the rule rather than the exception (van Loo et al., 2013). It may also be noted that such difficulties are relatively common in medical practice as well, even when signs (biomarkers) can be added to symptom descriptions. "Wrong diagnoses" are only discovered—if and when they are—through the wisdom of hindsight (Newman-Toker et al., 2020). It has been estimated that there are about twelve million wrong medical diagnoses made annually in the USA (Agha et al., 2022).

Some Reflections

One question of significance concerns the introduction of the term "diagnosis". Once again, we may guess that the choice of language is generated by the professional identity of the constructors, revealing a bias towards a medical perspective, making it more accessible and user-friendly for the medical profession. Unfortunately, the usage of language associated with the medical profession often produces associative misunderstandings, leading many to assume that the categories are medical/biological phenomena in nature and origin. Which is rather a shame, as it contradicts the explicit ideas that lie behind their creation, as we have noted.

To develop, formulate and deliver psychosocial interventions, we psychotherapists need a classification system just as much as medical doctors do. It is worthwhile noting that, working with couples and families, we also have a need of extra categories—we strive to identify communication patterns, relationship patterns and organizational patterns quickly, so that we can begin to consider what kind of intervention might be most helpful. An example is given in the chapter by Sheehan in this volume (see Chapter 2) where he describes a model for systemic practitioners to diagnose parental alienation. Importantly, while the diagnostic categories of DSM and ICD are created to be applied to the individual, couple and family therapists are trained to embrace a broader view, to explore not only the working of the individual mind, but also the network of relationships within which that mind exists— the relational and interactional context that binds the psychological and sociological domains together. Indeed, one limitation concerning the use of ICD/DMS is that, as they are individually focused, over-reliance on using them as a base for choosing interventions may encourage a kind of blindness to the significance of social factors as causal and maintaining factors in human suffering.

Belief in the utility and importance of the ICD/DSM has justified involving hundreds of thousands of professionals in their work with millions of patients, consuming enormous amounts of money in the process. The uncertainty of the categories and the individual syndromes is a challenge for both clinicians and researchers. But science must begin somewhere, and history tells us that mistakes made along the way are usually corrected sooner or later. However, there is a special challenge inherent in nature of the social sciences (and both DSM and ICD are essentially social science projects in their focus and methodology, albeit carried out under the aegis of the medical professional): we are often trapped in, and limited by, the recursive nature of language, lacking physical referents to which we can anchor our concepts and theories. Here we may perhaps be envious of our fellow scientists in physics or biology.

4. What are the consequences of their implementation? How well do they match the intended purpose?

The diagnostic systems are relatively simple, and it might seem reasonable to assume that there should be few problems with applying them. However, research informs us that attempts to implement an idea or method into an established organization are often more complicated in both theory and practice than the actual idea that is to be implemented (Fixsen et al., 2005; May, 2013). National health services are huge conglomerates that include many discrete units all established to pursue their own specialty. Also, private health services exist side by side with public utilities. According to implementation theory, there will be a tendency for each organization to absorb any new idea by adapting it into their own established way of thinking and working. Thus, the fact that medical doctors will use the categories as a precursor to begin appropriate and recommended medical treatment should be no surprise. In a parallel manner, psychotherapists may use the self-same categories to help them identify relevant therapeutic approaches: the category "depression" for example, will require a different kind of thinking than that of "ADHD".

To discuss whether the expressed purposes of the two diagnostic systems are being achieved would necessarily seem to rest upon the answers to two questions: firstly, have they been properly applied and secondly, does society benefit in terms of improved levels of health at the individual level?

Those responsible for both DSM and ICD seem to be pleased with the answer to the first question. The authors note that the systems are used on a broad, international scale by more and more practitioners—and not only doctors, but also by nurses, psychologists, psychotherapists, counsellors and educational professionals, amongst others. And being used by such professional groups, one may assume that generally they are being applied in ways that would meet the approval of the authors. There also seems a high degree of enthusiasm amongst insurance companies, politicians, civil servants and other officials who are responsible for organizing and allocating the finite resources of the health services. A clear and strict diagnostic procedure that also helps identify specific treatment is of great value to those who must organize and finance treatment services, simplifying many aspects of their work.

The data required to answer the second question—does the application of the system benefit the general health of the population—is more difficult to find a clear answer to (Collaborators, 2022). But in general terms, the answer at present would seem to be no: while there are many difficulties in measuring the incidence of mental illness over time, there is a general consensus that there is an increase, although by how much is uncertain (Richter et al., 2019) Explanations for this are potentially many, varied and complex, and there is no space to discuss them in detail here. Perhaps the most extreme critical perspective concerning the role and value of diagnostic systems is that if they are based on false premises about the nature of human emotional suffering, their application will probably not be very helpful (Braslow et al., 2020; Niv, 2021). This criticism is often connected to what might be called the medicalizing and biologizing of human emotional suffering (Slife et al., 2010). Suffice it to say, those who favour the diagnostic-treatment system can only hope that the apparent negative feedback thus far obtained is simply a temporary trend, due possibly to the way the system is applied and how the effects are evaluated. Other purposes, regarding the collection of data on course, morbidity, mortality and so on, are obviously facilitated by having a clear diagnostic coding system. But once again, the radical critics suggest that the information obtained by using the systems as guidelines is irretrievably flawed—for the simple reason that they are based on premises that do not accurately reflect the nature of human existence.

The answers to our two questions would therefore seem to be mixed: while the system is being applied more and more, with the help of more and more sophisticated instruments, positive results for the general population are doubtful (or at least unclear). What is clear is that a lot of statistical data is being collected and that much of the research in the field of mental health is anchored in the two systems.

Some Reflections

A systemic couple and family therapist will not always think in terms of individual diagnoses, as relationship categories such as conflict or crisis might be more appropriate. But whether introduced by the therapist ("Might I ask if you are feeling depressed?") or by the client ("I think my child might be autistic".) once an individual diagnosis is placed on the table, it can usually be weaved into the developing narrative of the systemic therapeutic process. As was noted earlier, no couple or family therapist can avoid using a system of categories, and at an individual level, and at the present time, the DSM/ICD system is the only game in town (even if there are several interesting competitors under development) that also has the benefit of connecting us to the dominant social and medical narratives (reflected in social praxis, laws and regulations), and thus may contribute to making life easier for the client in navigating the social system, as well as helping the therapist to search for relevant knowledge.

However, two ideas are of special concern for the CFT therapist, aware as she is of the power of sociological influences on the development of the individual: these are the ideas of the "normal brain" and the "normal mind".

In both psychiatry and in psychotherapy, there is often to be found an assumption that unwanted distress experienced by an individual (and/or that she causes in others) is a sign that "something" is wrong with her brain and/or mind. The logical assumption here is that if the individual's brain is functioning "normally" then the individual would not experience personal distress or cause it in others. This idea would seem to hold the promise that, in the distant future, science might develop the means to keep everyone's experience and behaviour within "normal" limits by, for example, balancing the biochemistry of the brain within specified, "normal" parameters and thereby relegating a great deal of distress to an imperfect past. This is indeed the logic behind, for example, the medical treatment of depression. Unfortunately, despite many years of trying, researchers have not been able to find evidence for such a premise (Moncrieff et al., 2022; Nour et al., 2022; Schmaal, 2022; Winter et al., 2022). The opposing paradigm is that the idea of the normal brain is a myth: rather, it is the nature of living organisms to produce biological variety as the central motor in the process of evolution, a perspective known as neurodiversity (Singer, 2019).

An isomorphic argument sometimes appears based on the idea of a "normal" mind. In this case, it assumes that if the individual thinks/lives/behaves in a "right" way, then the result will be that she will feel little distress and have few problems (e.g. in the case of CBT, see Craske, 2012, Ch. 2 & 3). This idea is the basis of many psychotherapeutic and medical interventions and is applied to many issues, from phobias to schizophrenia. There is of course the common observation that might appear to affirm this belief: when an individual approaches a therapist and asks for help, the pathway towards eventual relief of suffering is often the apparent result of learning to think or behave in different ways. But such an observation cannot be interpreted to mean that suffering was the consequence of thinking wrongly, or of not possessing a normal mind. For most of us, the journey through life presents a great many challenges, threats and unpleasant shocks. We cannot be prepared for all of them. If we judge people who find themselves unable to cope with distress, solve problems or manage pain as being unnormal or wrong, then it may very well lead us into the position of considering them as being comparatively less competent, weaker and even inferior—as lacking something that non-sufferers and good problem-solvers possess. Such thinking has shamed many sufferers, adding a double burden to their pain, an example of blaming the victim.

The history of ideas teaches us that both the idea and nature of the individual may constructively be viewed as social constructs, meaning that the thoughts, feelings and behaviours that individuals use to identify themselves and others are supported or hindered by the combined will and response of the social groups in which they live (Berger & Luckmann, 1966; Hacking, 1999; Sveinsdóttir, 2015). In attempting to understand human emotional suffering, we have suggested that any theoretical perspective that is based on only one of the three domains that are involved in the creation and maintenance of individual experience (the biological, the psychological or the sociological) will be incomplete. A pre-set belief used to identify and explain difference—for example, that emotional suffering is a question only of biology (or psychology, or sociology)—is not only truncated, but it may also be harmful. Truncated because all three domains are always involved in some way in the production of experience, and possibly harmful because ignoring up to two-thirds of what makes us human may produce a skewed understanding of the nature of suffering, leading to treatment interventions that may also be skewed. As with any other epistemological domain, the scope of human nature is so great that to try and understand it, we must begin by reducing its complexity and focusing on small pieces of it. But we should never forget that we have done so, thereby falling into the trap of believing that the cleaved part is the whole story—of mistaking an understanding of a part as constituting an explanation of the whole.

Labels that we use to describe ourselves or others are capable of being used either in a destructive or a constructive fashion, and this is just as true of everyday terms as it is of diagnostic labels, and observing communication patterns and how they are used to support or undermine others is a fundamental skill for a systemic therapist. While the implementation of ICD/DSM will not be a requirement of system-oriented psychotherapy as specified by its theory, it is easily integrated into its application where appropriate or necessary.

Final Reflection

The purpose of this chapter was to examine if systemic couple and family therapists can coexist with or even use the categories of ICD/DSM in our work, or if there are contradictions so great that it is neither possible nor desirable.

The three domains of biology, psychology and sociology are themselves categories: recognizing this starting point should ring warning bells, as the intellectual exercise of thinking of a human being as only biological, or only psychological or only sociological is based on an artificial distinction—necessary for the existence of the disciplines themselves, but hardly relevant for life itself. However, to study human beings at all, we need a methodology, we need a way to bring some semblance of order and we need to simplify. But there can be no excuse for mistaking the tools that we use to study the world for the world itself, or as Korzybsky (1933/1958) said: "the map is not the territory, and the name is not the thing named". We use categories to help bring order to our perception and to narrow our focus of study, but that order is not necessarily in the world: the world is not pre-packed into convenient boxes that have printed labels pasted on their sides informing us of the nature of the contents. However, as we noted in the beginning, one of the trickier and insidious aspects of using categories is that the more effective and helpful they prove to be, the more invisible they tend to become, until finally we may even forget about their existence and the roles that they play in organizing our cognition and perception (Bowker & Star, 2000). We may then make the error of thinking that the world really is the way that we have cognized it, forgetting about the mediating influence of the concepts we have used to guide and support our cognizing. We suggest that the two diagnostic systems are best seen as cognitive tools, not arbiters of reality, and when viewed as such they can help make our work simpler, and perhaps even better.

References

Agha, L., Skinner, J., & Chan, D. (2022). Improving efficiency in medical diagnosis. *JAMA, 327*(22), 2189–2190. https://doi.org/10.1001/jama.2022.8587

Allsopp, K., Read, J., Corcoran, R., & Kinderman, P. (2019). Heterogeneity in psychiatric diagnostic classification. *Psychiatry Research, 279*, 15–22. https://doi.org/10.1016/j.psychres.2019.07.005

Almeida, R. V., & Tubbs, C. Y. (2020). Intersectionality: A liberation-Based healing perspective. In K. S. Wampler, R. B. Miller, & R. B. Seedall (Eds.), *The handbook of systemic family therapy Vol. 1: The profession of systemic family therapy* (pp. 227–250). Wiley.

American Psychiatric Association. (2013). *Diagnostic and statistical manual of mental disorders* (5th ed.). American Psychiatric Publishing.

Berger, P. L., & Luckmann, T. (1966). *The social construction of reality: A treatise in the sociology of knowledge.* Penguin.

Bowker, G. C., & Star, S. L. (2000). *Sorting things out: Classification and its Consequences.* MIT Press.

Braslow, J. T., Brekke, J. S., & Levenson, J. (2020). Psychiatry's myopia—Reclaiming the social, cultural and psychological in the psychiatric gaze. *JAMA Psychiatry.* https://doi.org/10.1001/jamapsychiatry.2020.2722

Caspi, A., et al. (2020). Longitudinal assessment of mental health disorders and comorbidities across 4 decades among participants in the Dunedin birth cohort study. *JAMA Network Open, 3,* 203–221. https://doi.org/10.1001/jamanetworkopen.2020.3221

Cohen, H., & Lefebvre, C. (2005). Bridging the category divide. In H. Cohen & C. Lefebvre (Eds.), *Handbook of categorization in cognitive science* (pp. 2–15). Elsevier.

Collaborators, G. M. D. (2022). Global, regional, and national burden of 12 mental disorders in 204 countries and territories, 1990–2019: A systematic analysis for the Global burden of disease study. *The Lancet Psychiatry, 9*(2), 137–150. https://doi.org/10.1016/S2215-0366(21)00395-3

Craske, M. G. (2012). *Cognitive-behavioral therapy.* American Psychological Association.

Fiske, P. (2019). The lexical fallacy in emotional research: Mistaking vernacular words for psychological entities. *Psychological Review* (Online first publication). http://dx.doi.org/10.1037/rev0000174

Fixsen, D. L., Naoom, S. F., Blasé, K. A., Friedman, R. M., & Wallace, F. (2005). *Implementation research: A synthesis of the literature.* University of South Florida, Louis de la Parte Florida Mental Health Institute.

Goodrich, T. J., Rampage, C., Ellman, B., & Halstead, K. (1998). *Feminist family therapy: A casebook.* Norton.

Hacking, I. (1999). *The social construction of what?* Harvard.

Harnad, S. (2005). To cognize is to categorize: Cognition is categorization. In H. Cohen & C. Lefebvre (Eds.), *Handbook of categorization in cognitive science* (pp. 20–30). Elsevier.

Hickey, P. (2021). *How psychiatry turned general difficulties in adaption into "real illnesses just like diabetes".* https://madinamerica.com/2021/03/psychiatry-real-illnesses/

Hyman, S. E. (2010). The diagnosis of mental disorder: The problem of reification. *Annual Review of Clinical Psychology, 6*, 155–179. https://doi.org/10.1146/annurev.clinpsy.3.022806.091532

Jablensky, A. (2016). Psychiatric classifications: Validity and utility. *World Psychiatry, 15*, 26–31.

Kendler, K. S. (2022). Potential lessons for DSM from contemporary philosophy of science. *JAMA Psychiatry, 79*(2), 99–100. https://doi.org/10.1001/jamapsychiatry.2021.3559

Korzybsky, A. (1933/1958). *Science and sanity* (4th ed.). International Non-Aristotelian Library.

Lakoff, G. (1987). *Women, fire and dangerous things: What categories reveal about the mind*. University of Chicago Press.

May, C. (2013). Towards a general theory of implementation. *Implementation Science, 8*, 18. https://doi.org/10.1186/1748-5908-8-18

McGeorge, C. R., Walsdorf, A. A., Edwards, L. L., Benson, K. E., & Coburn, K. O. (2020). Sexual orientation and gender identity: Considerations for systemic therapists. In K. S. Wampler, R. B. Miller, & R. B. Seedall (Eds.), *The handbook of systemic family therapy. Vol. 1: The profession of systemic family therapy* (pp. 251–272). Wiley.

Medical News Today. (June 2021). *Gender bias in medical diagnosis*. https://www.medicalnewstoday.com

Medical News Today. (October 2021). *What to know about gender bias in healthcare*. https://www.medicalnewstoday.com

Moncrieff, J., Cooper, R. E., Stockmann, T., Amendola, S., Hengartner, M. P., & Horowitz, M. A. (2022). The serotonin theory of depression: A systematic umbrella review of the evidence. *Molecular Psychiatry*. Published online on July 20, 2022. https://doi.org/10.1038/s41380-022-01661-0

Newman-Toker, D. E., Wang, Z., Zhu, Y., Nassery, N., Saber Tehrani, A. S., Schaffer, A. C., Yu-Moe, C. W., Clemens, G. D., Fanai, M., & Siegel, D. (2020). Rate of diagnostic errors and serious misdiagnosis-related harms for major vascular events, infections, and cancers: Toward a national incidence estimate using the "Big Three." *Diagnosis, 8*, 67–84. https://doi.org/10.1515/dx-2019-0104

Niv, J. (2021). The primacy of behavioral research for understanding the Brain. *Behavioral Neuroscience, 135*(5), 601–609. https://doi.org/10.1037/bne0000471

Nour, M. M., Liu, Y., & Dolan, R. J. (2022). Functional neuroimaging in psychiatry and the case for failing better. *Neuron, 110*, 2524–2544. https://doi.org/10.1016/j.neuron.2022.07.005

Onnis, L. (2016). From pragmatics to complexity: Developments and perspectives of systemic psychotherapy. In M. Borcsa & P. Stratton (Eds.), *Origins and originality in family therapy and systemic practice* (pp. 13–23). European Family Therapy Association Series. Springer, Cham. https://doi.org/10.1007/978-3-319-39061-1_2

Plana-Ripoli, O., et al. (2019). Exploring comorbidity within mental disorders among a danish national population. *JAMA Psychiatry, 76*(3), 259–270. https://doi.org/10.1001/jamapsychiatry.2018.3658

Raskin, J. D. (2018). What might an alternative to the DSM suitable for psychotherapists look like? *Journal of Humanistic Psychology, 1*–8. https://doi.org/10.1177/0022167818761919

Richter, D., Wall, A., Bruen, A., & Whittington, R. (2019). Is the global rate of adult mental health increasing? Systematic review and meta-analysis. *Acta Psychiatrica Scandinavica.* https://doi.org/10.1111/acps.13083

Schmaal, L. (2022). The search for clinically useful neuroimaging markers of depression a worthwhile pursuit or a futile quest? *JAMA Psychiatry, 79*(9), 845–846. https://doi.org/10.1001/jamapsychiatry.2022.1606

Singer, J. (2019). Reflections on the neurodiversity movement 20 years on. In *Neurodiversity: 20th anniversary of the birth of the concept: Advocacy for positive recognition of human diversity and its future.* https://www.etsy.com/ca-fr/listing/701221413/neurodiversity-20th-anniversary-of-the??

Slife, B. D., Burchfield, C., & Hedges, D. (2010). Interpreting the "biologization" of psychology. *Journal of Mind and Behavior, 31*(3–4), 165–177.

Sveinsdóttir, Á. (2015). Social construction. *Philosophy Compass, 10*(12), 884–892. https://doi.org/10.1111/phc3.12265

van Loo, H. M., Romeijn, J. W., de Jonge, P., & Schoevers, R. A. (2013). Psychiatric comorbidity and causal disease models. *Preventive Medicine, 57*(6), 748–752. https://doi.org/10.1016/j.ypmed.2012.10.018

Wakefield, J. C. (1992). Disorder as harmful dysfunction: A conceptual critique of DSM-III-R's definition of mental disorder. *Psychological Review, 99*(2), 232–247. https://doi.org/10.1037/0033-295X.99.2.232

Walters, M., Carter, C., Papp, P., & Silverstein, O. (1988). *The invisible web.* Guilford.

Werkhoven, S. (2021). Natural kinds of mental disorder. *Synthese, 199,* 10135–10165. https://doi.org/10.1007/s11229-021-03239-9

Winter, N. R., Leenings, R., Ernsting, J., Sarink, K., Fisch, L., Emden, D., & Hahn, T. (2022). Quantifying deviations of brain structure and function in major depressive disorder across neuroimaging modalities. *JAMA Psychiatry, 79*(9), 879–888. https://doi.org/10.1001/jamapsychiatry.2022.1780

World Health Organization. (1992). *ICD-10: The ICD classification of mental and behavioural disorders: Clinical descriptions and diagnostic guidelines.* WHO.

World Health Organization. (1993). *ICD-10: The ICD classification of mental and behavioural Disorders: Diagnostic criteria for research.* WHO.

Zachar, P., & Kendler, K. S. (2017). The philosophy of nosology. *Annual Review of Clinical Psychology, 13,* 49–71. https://doi.org/10.1146/annurev-clinpsy-032816-045020

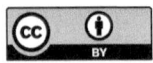

8

"The Challenges Will Remain": Systemic Work with Families of Children Needing Extra Care

Halvor de Flon and Jim Sheehan

Introduction

After working as a systemic therapists in many different contexts over the several decades, it is our observation that systemic family therapy is often associated with an understanding and expectation that problems and challenges in families and family living can and should be solved and forced to disappear with the help of various kinds of systemic interventions. Most models of family therapy and systemic work include an understanding of how problems develop within systems and how therapists can help the system to act in ways that make them disappear. Across the same time period, the systemic field has broadened in its conception of itself, and this broadening is nowhere more evident than through the introduction of the term 'systemic work'. Systemic work

H. de Flon (✉) · J. Sheehan
Department of Family Therapy and Systemic Practice, Faculty of Social
Studies, Oslo, Norway
e-mail: halvor.flon@vid.no

© The Author(s) 2024
S. M. Myra et al. (eds.), *New Horizons in Systemic Practice with Children
and Families*, Palgrave Texts in Counselling and Psychotherapy,
https://doi.org/10.1007/978-3-031-38111-9_8

129

is the term now used to depict professional practice in many different kinds of working contexts such as child protection services, kindergartens and schools (see Chapter 7 by Axberg and Petitt, this volume, and Chapter 10 by van Roosmalen, this volume). This chapter will concentrate on systemic work with families with children that have different and various kinds of difficulties that they have had since birth or as a result of accidents and injuries. The children in the families we are focusing on here have one thing in common, namely they all suffer from chronic or long-lasting conditions. An incomplete list of such conditions includes severe Diabetes, Autism Spectrum Disorder (ASD), Attention Deficit Hyperactivity Disorder (ADHD), Tourette's Syndrome, Down's syndrome, Developmental Disability, physical injuries or other conditions seen as incurable. A further common factor is that the families are in contact with many different services within the helping system such as specialists within hospitals, social welfare services of different kinds and institutions that provide "relief" and practical help and support. The task for services involved can be a combination of assessment and treatment with respect to the different conditions connected to a specific syndrome, sickness or injury and the provision of different kinds of support. What has been missing historically for these families in the Norwegian context, is a service that provides parental and family guidance and support to cope with a situation that is and probably will be affected by the conditions mentioned above and their consequences for the foreseeable future. The common factor for most of these families is that they have daily challenges that must be solved daily and that such challenges will not disappear or go away. The challenges will change, but they will almost always remain in one way or another.

Families in such situations often experience that the different parts of the helping systems they are in contact with cooperate poorly and that they, as parents, must be the bridge between them. This "job" often takes a lot of time and resources from parents who are already in a situation that demands great effort from them in taking care of the daily needs of the child who needs extra care and the needs of that child's siblings. The individual agencies that together make up the overall helping system mostly offer help of high quality but users often experience them as poorly coordinated and fragmented (Rogne, 2016).

Overburdened parents find that they must compensate for the deficits in coordination between services by functioning additionally as a kind of infrastructure of information between services. An example of this kind of additional demand arises from the fact that helping and school systems are often organized by age—categories which means that families must live with the fact that they often have to say goodbye to helpers and teachers when their child reaches a certain age and to establish new relations with a new set of helpers.

In presenting this chapter within a volume on 'new horizons' within systemic therapy and practice, we wish to emphasize two matters. The first concerns the newly evolving recognition of this arena of systemic practice as a specialism in its own right. No longer regarded as a field of practice where the novice practitioner may dip in and out to learn and practice discrete systemic skills with a client group who will 'always be there', work with families where children suffer with chronic conditions must now be viewed as a practice domain that demands a very broad range of systemic skills made available in the service of the whole family and its constituent parts in addition to the performance of these skills as part of a co-ordinating function aimed at enhancing the connectedness of the family's helping system as a whole, thus unburdening parents and children from a responsibility they should not, but often do, have to bear. The second matter is a consequence of the first. Because the work involves a type of systemic practice operating on many different levels simultaneously, it offers the experienced practitioner entry to a highly complex social field wherein new and unexpected opportunities for professional and personal development abound.

Our purpose in this chapter is to describe a variety of systemic practices with families with children that need extra care and where these family and child challenges will probably remain in some way or another. How can we characterize good systemic interventions in such family contexts? What do these interventions look like? We will also try to describe the systemic interventions that are responsive to the challenges arising from the poorly coordinated systems of help that surround these families.

The experiences this chapter is built on have their origin in a service established and developed in a middle-sized Norwegian city where the main task of the service is to support the families described. The service is called "the family – guidance service." The first author has worked in this service in the past and remains connected to it. The remainder of the chapter will be organized in the following way: following a description of the family-guidance service three family vignettes will be described in addition to the systemic work that was performed with each of the three families. This will allow the reader to receive a rich description of a small sample of systemic practices/interventions that respond to a highly differentiated arena of families with children that need additional care of one kind or another. The reader will also be invited to note the many different, and often competing, theoretical frameworks that underpin the rich variety of practices that comprise this area of systemic work. The vignettes will be followed by a reflection upon the shape of the thera-peutic relationship in this area of work with additional attention being paid to the support required for this key relationship at the heart of the practice.

The Family-guidance Service

The family-guidance service (FGS) began in 2018 and the main purpose of the service was to support families with children with special needs with guidance and supervision as an addition to practical help. According to Norwegian law, local municipal authorities are obliged to give parents with children that have special needs guidance in how to cope with their situation. The content of the guidance is not defined in the law, but traditionally such service has been seen as experts giving practical advice about "how to do it" by educating care—givers on how to cope with different kind of challenges such as aggression, sleeping prob-lems, school—refusal and so on. The FGS was initially designed to do something else but their function was not clearly defined or described.

How to organize a new service, and where to place it within a larger organisational framework is always an important issue that needs thorough consideration. In this municipality, the provision of health and social services is organized in a way that people that need help apply for this to a central unit. Case-managers assess the application and decide what the individual or family will be offered. In this process, the case-manager usually collects information by interviewing the person or persons that have applied, considers their requests against the background of usual service responses and subsequently discusses with colleagues and leaders what might be reasonable to offer. The assessment could then be discussed with the applying person(s) but not always. The process and the decision is based on the "Law of health and social services" and is always communicated in written form. The decision is sent to the person and to the municipal service that would carry out the delivery of the service response. What was experienced in the earlier phases of the FGS was that there was often a kind of "gap" between what the case-managers and their leaders considered as good enough help and what the receiving persons' experience was of the help offered. The FGS was organizationally located among the case-managers who assigned work directly to the FGS staff.

When this service was started it was a key-point of its foundation that families' descriptions and stories about what they felt they needed should be one of the pillars or cornerstones in the working relation between the family and the therapist. It was also decided that the service should be based on a systemic understanding that implies seeing human behaviour and all phenomena in context (Bateson, 1972). This also implies a relational view of life which means that what's happening between people is the therapist's central focus. But now, I will turn to the three vignettes. Each vignette depicts a child and parents facing unique challenges associated with a particular chronic condition and tells the story of how the FGS tried to help them and their response to this help.

Advocacy as a Systemic Intervention: Gabriel and His Mother Claire

Gabriel is a boy of 11 living with his mother and with no contact with his father in the last 5 years. He has two grown up sisters living in another part of the country. Gabriel's mother has not been able to work for the last two years due to health problems including a condition of severe fatigue. She has now very a small income support from the social welfare office through decisions made for 6 months at a time. Gabriel is diagnosed with Autism Spectrum Disorder (ASD). He started school when he was 6 years old, but after 6 months it was almost impossible for him to be at school more than one or two days a week and then maybe only up to an hour at a time. This has been the situation since. He is now attending the unit within his class designed for pupils with ASD struggling with coming to and staying at school. One of the goals for him at school is that he should be at school for about three hours every schoolday, but quite often he does not manage to come to school more than once a week and for some weeks not at all. His mother use to drive him and follow him into the classroom. Many efforts had been made to try to improve the situation. The role of the "family guidance service" was to offer Gabriel's mother Claire guidance sessions and one of the purposes of this offer was to help Claire to help Gabriel to come to school more often. Claire said yes to this offer although she also said she did not have very high expectations regarding the usefulness of this. She also told the therapists after a while that she had felt that there was no option to say no.

In the first session, we talked about Gabriel and her history, and she told us that she was exhausted after years of worries and uncertainty. Duncan (2014) proposes that agreement between therapist and client about goals is important in order to succeed and be helpful. Based on that we started to make a list of what worried her in order to sort out what topics she perhaps wanted to focus. It soon became clear that what worried her most was her economic situation. She had not been able to work for many years due to her physical condition and the family situation and she no longer had a right to be reported sick from her doctor which meant that she had to rely for her income on social welfare who made decisions about financial support for three months ahead. The amount of aid was limited, and Claire had to be very careful about what she used money on. She also said that she, through the clinic that had assessed and treated Gabriel, had participated in courses and other kind of psychoeducational activities and she thought that she had a good grip on what ASD is or could be and how this affected Gabriel and herself. She knew when she could push him a bit more in order to help him go to school or participate in social events in the family, such as birthdays, Christmas and so on and when she could not. She did not feel the need for more education and advice on how to cope with the situation and she also felt that the helping systems questioned her competence and that this was an additional burden.

We then talked about how she thought or wished the family-guidance service could assist her. She said that she really did not know and that she had said yes to come to talk with us mostly because she felt that she had to say yes. We talked about how we (FGS) could be a resource for her and Gabriel and not an additional work task that could turn into an extra burden. Would it be of any help if we also met Gabriel? Should we have the sessions at their home with them both? Did she want us to experience alongside her how she and Gabriel interacted in challenging situations? Claire said no to these suggestions, and after a while she said that she felt what was most stressful to her was her income situation, which she assumed we could not help her with. Minuchin (1991) criticized post-modern and social constructionist-oriented family therapy for seducing people to believe that problems could be dissolved (and solved) in language by developing a different way of talking about what is challenging. Sundet (2009) points out the importance of the therapist's willingness to support their clients also in practical ways, such as using their authority to impact the client's essential life conditions. As a therapist in this situation, I thought it would be of limited help for the family to talk to me about how stressful it is to not know how much money they had at their disposal the following month. This would hardly help and certainly would not solve the problem or create a more predictable income situation. This challenge is a part of the context (Bateson, 1972), and a systemic therapist should always be aware of the conditions under which their clients live and be ready to help them with these in so far as they can.

In this situation, I asked Claire for permission to talk to her case-manager in the social welfare department about her situation and to spell out how her circumstances affected her ability to be a mother to a son that really needed much input from his surroundings. She said yes to this and I made contact with the case-manager and pointed out that working on parental skills which requires a lot of psychological effort is a very different task when you are stressed about your basic life conditions. The case-manger understood this and made a formal decision on financial support within a longer time horizon. For Claire, this meant less concern and stress and a better capacity to withstand demanding situations together with Gabriel.

Gabriel showed a lot of anxiety in transitional situations in general (leaving home for school) and in social situations including with persons he doesn't know. These feelings could often overwhelm him and force him to stay at home instead of going to school. Anxiety and other affective disorders have been reported as co-morbid conditions to ASD (Hudson et al., 2017; van Steensel et al., 2013). In addition, a higher level of attachment difficulties are also reported in children with ASD in contrast with comparable groups (Naber et al., 2007; van Ijzendoorn et al., 2007). These feelings could often overwhelm him and force him to stay at home instead of going to school. In such situation, he really needs his caregivers to offer a secure base. Dallos and Vetere (2009, 2014) describes how concepts from attachment theory as secure base (Bowlby, 1988) may be applied in systemic approaches. To be this secure base in challenging situations when Gabriel is overwhelmed by anxiety and other difficult feelings, he needs Claire to remain "strong" and capable of accommodating and containing his anxiety. Through theoretical and practical training, systemic practitioners will be aware of the influence of context on people's life and their possibilities to effect changes (de Flon, 2019b). In the case of Gabriel and Claire, we see that the material conditions have a significant impact on their situation. Duncan et al. (2010) claim that as much as 40% of the impact/outcome of therapeutic process is determined by factors outside the therapy, in other words, by what happens in the course of people living their everyday lives. In this case, it was necessary for the systemic therapist to be an advocate on behalf of the family in order to foster better possibilities for Claire to focus on her role and position as a caregiver for Gabriel. Sundet (2009) suggests in his research that the alliance between the family and the therapist becomes strengthened by a therapist's efforts to help with practical or material matters. This could mean writing letters of recommendation to social service or other services, adopting an advocacy role in meetings or making direct contact with other parts of the family's helping system.

This requires that practitioners take a position that secures a broad view of the family's context including their basic living conditions and show a capacity and willingness to expand the arena for systemic intervention to also include the professional system.

Parental Conflict Resolution as Systemic Intervention: Peter and His Parents

Peter is 15 years old and lives with his parents Johnny and June. Their municipal case-manager contacted the FGS and asked if we could have some sessions with June. In the first session, she told us that Peter was diagnosed with ASD and Attention Deficit Hyperactivity Disorder (ADHD) and that the family were experiencing severe challenges and that she would like us to talk with the whole family. We, therefore, decided to meet in their house and asked that both her husband and Peter would be at home. Peter said initially at the first session that it was not his first choice to start the day talking to a therapist but he could do it if we all could speak English in the session. His parents had already told me that he preferred English also at home with them and in school. Both his parents have other languages than Norwegian as their first languages, but they do not share the same first language. I said that was OK, but in my inner conversation with myself I was quite pessimistic about how I could perform as a family therapist in English. But I thought this was one way to try to build an alliance with Peter so I jumped into it. In my inner conversation, I also had Duncan (2014) in mind who maintains that therapists should be flexible in their work in order to achieve contact and build a working alliance with the client. One of the main characteristics of ASD is challenges with language (Reindal et al., 2023). I also knew that these challenges with language could be of many different kinds. Against this background as well I thought it was the right thing to follow his wish. In the session, it soon became clear that his parents often had opposite opinions about almost everything and that their communication was characterized by a mutual specification of each other in negative ways and by raised voices against each other. This obviously bothered Peter, and after a while he left the table where we were seated and moved down onto the floor and found a place to sit by his cat that had been sleeping in the corner of the room. He started to comfort the cat, and the cat seemed to like it. I then asked him what he thought about the conversation so far and what he thought would be helpful for the family. He then said; "both the cat and I would have a better life if the two of them (pointing to the parents) could stop arguing and treating each other like crap." This was a powerful statement and the parents stopped arguing and looked rather sad and surprised. I used the moment to ask them how they felt about what Peter just said. Johnny said that he was not aware of the strength of his son's feelings about how he and his wife communicated. "He is always in his room gaming on his computer, and I really did not know that he had heard so much of our arguing." June said that she knew very well and thought it was very strange that Johnny did not know. Johnny reacted to this and soon their arguing was speeding up again. "Now you can see for yourself" Peter said. "They cannot stop, and it is really bothering me a lot because they are arguing almost always about me – it is not cool to be reminded that I am such a burden to them." Both parents said to him that he was not a burden, but I think he did not believe them. I then suggested that the next sessions should be without Peter to give the parents an opportunity to work on their relationship.

This case focused on the importance of the therapist's ability to be flexible in their work with families with children that need extra care (Sheehan, 2020). The original request from this family was to help the family to communicate better. When the parents showed that they could not hold their conflict away from Peter, and he told the therapist very clearly that he was much bothered by the way they treated each other, it was important for the therapist to be flexible enough to change the focus from finding the right language in which the whole family could communicate and engage with him to assisting the parents with conflict resolution techniques to be applied to the area of their parenting of Peter.

Harnessing Family Resources: Taylor, Her Mother and Extended Family

Taylor is a 9-year-old girl who has been through several brain surgeries because of a severe epileptic condition. Assessment has shown that her cognitive function is that of a 5-year-old child. Managing her medication is challenging because her epilepsy is unstable and unpredictable. Her cognitive function is affected by the epilepsy and the medication. Assessment of her epilepsy has shown that she gets small seizures several times a day which are not always possible to recognize, even for her mother. The seizures can be observed as small periods of "vanishing."

Early in the contact with the family Taylor's mother spoke about her struggle to convince her family about Taylor's condition. She said that she experienced them as having various ways of overlooking her challenges and expecting too much of her. This could often lead to difficult situations where, for example, one of Taylor's aunts or her grandfather, made too excessive demands or expectations of her. This often led to conflict between Taylor and her relatives which greatly concerned Andrea, Taylor's mother. Lately, Taylor was refusing to be looked after by anyone other than her mother. Andrea really needed the respite her relatives could offer, but in the current situation they were not in a position to be the resources she desperately needed.

A systemic therapist working with families with children needing extra care and with challenges that in some ways will remain has to be able to work in many ways and on many different levels (de Flon, 2019a) In this situation, the therapist suggested convening the family, inspired by the concept of family conference groups (Frost et al., 2014). The intention with this intervention is to harness the family resources in order to move towards a more unified understanding of Taylor and her needs. In the gathering Andrea, her sister and her partner and 3 grandparents participated. The therapist proceeded by speaking about the intention for the meeting and gave a summary of Taylor's condition based on the assessment and the consequences for her and her functioning. This "teaching" or psychoeducation of the family is a way of creating a common base for exchange of experiences and knowledge about Taylor. This "teaching" was followed up with an interview with

Andrea about Taylor and what she as her mother needed from the family while the other family members where listening. The conversation was organized as a kind of reflecting team (Andersen, 1991; de Flon, 2017), giving the family opportunity to comment on what they had heard. In the following conversation, the family expressed surprise at hearing about Taylor's cognitive level and how the epilepsy affects her behaviour. This knowledge and Andrea's expression of her needs connected to being a parent for Taylor triggered a conversation about how they could be helpful. This led to a better situation for Taylor and Andrea and the family started a process becoming more like a team trying to achieve the same goals.

The Therapeutic Relationship and Its Support

Building and maintaining the therapeutic relationship with parents and children in families 'where challenges remain' poses many of its own challenges for systemic therapists no matter how experienced such practitioners might be. It often means entering a relational field where parents already feel let down by, and distrustful of, outside services who they feel do not comprehend the magnitude of the daily tasks they face in caring for their child. Indeed, when coming face-to-face with the enormity of demands falling naturally on the parents of children with very serious and unremitting physical and psychological conditions, the first reaction experienced by the practitioner may be a desire to run in the opposite direction as fast as they can. While wanting to build trust with parents and children, they may be met initially by a very hesitant parental response allied to a cynicism regarding the meaningfulness of a professional presence in their lives.

The systemic practitioner needs to have patience with the trust building process which may only progress through repeated engagement and often enduring together repeated failure in the shared efforts to bring about some degree of amelioration in the family's situation. The irony is that client trust in the therapist may only evolve out of an experience of the professional's authentic efforts to assist and to go on trying to assist in contexts where a pattern of 'one step forward followed by two steps backwards' seems to be the norm. There is something about the process of the professional's exposure to the intensity of child demands upon parents and their daily confrontation with unsolvable problems that builds a unique form of professional-parent solidarity over time. Alongside patience, the systemic practitioner needs the capacity to witness the prolonged and enduring suffering of both parents and children. Witnessing always involves a capacity to *listen* carefully to the experiences of parents but also involves a willingness to *see* first-hand some of the different predictable daily crises that the care of their children presents. An empathic kind of witnessing involves engaging as deeply as one can with the enduring suffering of parents before returning to oneself with the realization that 'this could have been me'.

The therapeutic relationship in families where challenges remain also requires a flexibility on the part of the practitioner. While many therapeutic meetings may happen in the professional's office while the child is either at school or being cared for elsewhere, the relationship will often require that some meetings happen in the family home and some of these meetings may need to happen as part of a response to an unforeseen crisis which occurs outside of normal working hours. An adaptable, flexible positioning on the part of the systemic therapist is part of what assists with the continuous building of a trusting client-professional relationship where the clients experience the authentic, heart-filled and caring engagement of the practitioner.

Working with such parents and family situations can be very demanding for professionals. It is not unusual for practitioners to shrink back from situations when confronted with the enormity of what a parent and child may be experiencing. They may try to persuade their supervisor that the case should be closed as nothing can be achieved or they may come up with some reasons why the work should be passed on from themselves to another practitioner. Or they may feel assaulted within by intolerable feelings of guilt and abandonment as they leave behind a distressed parent and a screaming child on a Friday evening on the way to meet their own partner and children for a pizza on the same evening. While it is inevitable that some therapeutic relationships have to end for a myriad of different reasons, the needs of most families in contexts where 'the challenges remain' are better fulfilled when their therapists also 'remain'. However, for therapists to find the capacity to not only remain but remain in an active, engaged, empathic and dependable positioning in their relationship with families they need a level of support that does justice to the nature of their own challenge. This means having a regular, dependable and engaged relationship with a trusted supervisor who knows the territory of the practitioner's work. It means having a supervisor who can 'hold' the practitioner as they grapple with the many complex emotions that may be aroused in the process of witnessing the intense suffering of others where such suffering is likely to find no real abatement other than small levels of transformation flowing from the experience of solidarity that joins the client family, the systemic therapist and their supervisor. It is also important for the practitioner or the therapist to be part of a supportive systems of colleagues to discuss, reflect and share joys and challenges connected to their work.

Conclusion

The purpose of this chapter has been to demonstrate both the utility and complexity of the systemic practices that address the situation where families need support in contexts where they have children with chronic conditions who need extra care and where no end to the challenges comes into view. The chapter has highlighted just a small sample of the systemic skills deployed by practitioners in this service arena. Another aim in writing this chapter has been to give further recognition to this domain of systemic practice as a specialism in its own right. The complexity of the territory offers itself to either the novice or experienced practitioner as a ground rich with possibilities for personal and professional growth and development. At the centre of the work lies the therapeutic relationship where trust must often be built slowly and patiently through a series of trials, setbacks and provisional successes. The role of the supervisory relationship has also been characterized as a critical support for the many roles and functions performed by the practitioner.

References

Andersen, T. (1991). *The reflecting team: Dialogues and dialogues about the dialogues.* Norton.

Bateson, G. (1972). *Steps to an ecology of mind.* Ballentine Books.

Bowlby, J. (1988). *A secure base.* Basic Books.

Dallos, R., & Vetere, A. (2009). *Systemic therapy and attachment narratives: Applications in a range of clinical settings.* Routledge/Taylor & Francis Group.

Dallos, R., & Vetere, A. (2014). *Attachment narrative therapy: Patterns, stories and connection.* www.acamh.org/knowledge/articles/attachment-narrative-therapy-patterns-stories-and-connections

de Flon, H. (2017). The reflecting team approach: Different uses in live supervision and group supervision with both family therapy trainees and practitioners. In A. Vetere & J. Sheehan (Eds.), *Supervision of family therapy and systemic practice* (pp. 107–120). Springer International Publishing.

de Flon, H. (2019a). Hva er familieterapi? [What is family therapy]. In L. Lorås & O. Ness (Eds.), *Håndbok i familieterapi [Handbook in family therapy]* (pp. 15–24). Fagbokforlaget.

de Flon, H. (2019b). Hvordan blir man familieterapeut? [How to become a family therapist]. In L. Lorås & O. Ness (Eds.), *Håndbok i familieterapi [Handbook in family therapy]* (pp. 41–47). Fagbokforlaget.

Duncan, B. L. (2014). *On becoming a better therapist: Evidence-based practice one client at a time* (2nd ed.). American Pschological Association.

Duncan, B. L., Miller, S. D., Wampold, B. E., & Hubble, M. A. (2010). *The heart and soul of change: Delivering what works in therapy* (2nd ed.). American Psychological Association.

Frost, N., Abram, F., & Burgess, H. (2014). Family group conferences: Evidence, outcomes and future research. *Child & Family Social Work, 19*(4), 501–507.

Hudson, M., Dallos, R., & McKenzie, R. (2017). Systemic-attachment formulation for families of children with autism. *Advances in Autism, 3*(3), 142–153.

Minuchin, S. (1991). The seduction of constructivism. *Family Therapy Networker, 15,* 47–51.

Naber, F. B., Swinkels, S. H., Buitelaar, J. K., Bakermans-Kranenburg, M. J., van IJzendoorn, M. H., Dietz, C., van Daalen, H., & van Engeland, H. (2007). Attachment in toddlers with autism and other developmental disorders. *Journal of Autism and Developmental Disorders, 37*(6), 1123–1138.

Reindal, L., Nærland, T., Weidle, B., Lydersen, S., Andreassen, O. A., & Sund, A. M. (2023). Structural and pragmatic language impairments in children evaluated for Autism Spectrum Disorder (ASD). *Journal of Autism and Developmental Disorders, 53*(2), 701–719.

Rogne, K. T. (2016). I det lange løp - En oppfølgingsstudie om hverdagsliv og samliv i familier med utviklingshemmede barn. *Fokus På Familien, 44*(3), 220–239.

Sheehan, J. (2020). Couples with chronic illness: Challenges and opportunities in the long-term therapeutic relationship. In A. Vetere & J. Sheehan (Eds.), *Long term systemic therapy: Individuals, couples and families* (pp. 21–40). Springer International Publishing.

Sundet, R. (2009). *Client directed, outcome informed therapy in an intensive family therapy unit: A study of the use of research generated knowledge in clinical practice* (Dissertation, Department of Psychology, University of Oslo).

van Ijzendoorn, M. H., Rutgers, A. H., Bakermans-Kranenburg, M. J., Swinkels, S. H., van Daalen, E., Dietz, C., Nabler, F. B., Buitelaar, J. K., & van Engeland, H. (2007). Parental sensitivity and attachment in children with autism spectrum disorder: Comparison with children with mental retardation, with language delays, and with typical development. *Child Development, 78*(2), 597–608.

van Steensel, F. J., Bögels, S. M., & de Bruin, E. I. (2013). Psychiatric comorbidity in children with autism spectrum disorders: A comparison with children with ADHD. *Journal of Child and Family Studies, 22*(3), 368–376.

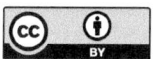

9

A Systemic Approach to School-Based Consultation: Combining Interventions That Belong to Different Theoretical Traditions

Ulf Axberg and Bill Petitt

In this chapter, we assume that the adoption of a systems perspective encourages—even requires—the possession of a plurality of theories and instruments because of the extremely complex nature of dynamic systems. To illustrate this idea, we describe how two separate intervention models, each derived from very different philosophical and theoretical traditions, have successfully been included within a single, systems-oriented framework. We describe a real-life, school-based intervention that combines a normative approach (Marte Meo), with a non-normative perspective (Coordination Meetings). The choice of models was made because of our understanding of the systems involved (individual, family,

U. Axberg (✉)
Department of Family Therapy and Systemic Practice, Faculty of Social Studies, VID Specialized University, Oslo, Norway
e-mail: ulf.axberg@vid.no

B. Petitt
Logos AB, Lerdala, Sweden
e-mail: bill.petitt@telia.com

S. M. Myra et al. (eds.), *New Horizons in Systemic Practice with Children and Families*, Palgrave Texts in Counselling and Psychotherapy,
https://doi.org/10.1007/978-3-031-38111-9_9

organization) and the goal of the intervention. This implies that the actual choice of models selected for this intervention (or indeed any intervention) can be thought of as being arbitrary. This thinking fits with the primary goal with this chapter, which is not to promote a specific intervention, but rather to illustrate the idea that a systems perspective can encompass any idea that helps increase our understanding and effectiveness.

Introduction

Sonny, an eight-year-old boy is described by his classroom teacher as hard to understand, and she and other staff members are beginning to experience his behaviour as tiresome, as are his peers at school. According to the teacher, he often explodes in anger, "Like a bolt from the blue". Furthermore, he isn't keeping up with the lessons and is also having more and more difficulties in contact with peers. They are starting to avoid him and exclude him from play, and she recently found out that they no longer invite him to their birthday parties. At times, he seeks contact with her, comes with various questions or shows things he has brought from home, but sadly enough often at inappropriate times—when she cannot respond properly to what he is showing or asking. The teacher has tried to talk to Sonny's mother about his problems and has recommended her to seek help from Child Psychiatry or the Social Services, but she finds it difficult to reach her. Sonny's mother says that the school is overly critical of him and that they exaggerate the problems. She thinks that Sonny must just be given time to mature. The father and mother are separated and he lives elsewhere, and the teacher has not been able to speak to him about Sonny's school situation.

The creation of the intervention that was finally named "*Marte Meo and Coordination Meetings (MAC)*" was a response to the realization that—over a period of time—certain children and their families repeatedly appeared as "cases" in different settings (such as the education system, Psychiatric Services, Social Services, and other related agencies). Closer examination of these cases seemed to reveal a common pattern. Quite often, the first occasion when the family was brought to official attention was soon after the child had started school, when the teachers noted that the child seemed to be experiencing difficulties in adaption in the classroom. There is a certain logic to this, as teachers daily meet children of the same age in groups and are thus in very special position to identify children whose behaviour deviates from generally accepted social parameters. The teachers did what they could to help in the school, of course, but if this failed to work, then often there followed a discussion in which the staff typically examined hypotheses about what the "cause" of the child's difficulties might be. Such hypotheses were usually focussed on factors that were external to the school—the family, possible psychiatric diagnoses and so on.

The next step in the pattern was that the school usually tried to involve the parents. If the desired results were still not forthcoming—if the parents wouldn't or couldn't help—then the school would suggest seeking expert help for the child, referring to their hypotheses to motivate this suggestion. Some parents declined to seek help as they did not feel that they had a problem at home, pointing out that their child only had problems at school and therefore they should be dealt with there. Other parents accepted the offered referral. However, in both cases, the result was often that the child's behaviour in school did not change—which could then lead to more suggestions for new referrals with still more services and experts. From the moment that the school first took contact with them, it also emerged as part of the pattern that it was easy for parents to feel that they were being criticized, particularly if they experienced the child's behaviour as being unproblematic in the home. If this happened, then they would tend to become defensive and critical of teachers and the pre-school/school. When this happened, there was a risk of a self-reinforcing, problem-affirming system of communicative behaviour developing around the child, in which both parts (family and school) felt blamed by the other. In turn, this generated the risk of an "epistemic breakdown", in which mutual distrust replaces mutual trust (Talia et al., 2021; Thayer, 1972). When this happens, it will often effectively hinder the establishment of a cooperative relationship—of building a working alliance to help the child. If such a relational context becomes established, this may also put an additional and even heavy burden on the child, as he is the nexus point between the home and school and it is he who will have to balance the conflicting relationships and the different sets of expectations they represent (Aponte, 1976). This may place the child in a particularly vulnerable and difficult position.

The Development of MAC

In response to this analysis, Ingegerd Wirtberg,[1] attached to the Department of Psychology at Lund University, took the initiative to establish a research project aimed at the first step in the pattern described above: how to intervene at the very first stage—when the teachers say that they have spotted a child who has difficulties in adapting to the culture of the classroom. The first stage of the project involved a research team and a group of professionals who would help develop and apply the intervention. It was located in the county of Skövde, an area in which Ingegerd already had a professional network established over many years of teaching and supervising there. It was this project that resulted in the school-based intervention that later came to be named *Marte Meo and Coordination Meetings (MAC)* (Axberg et al., 2006). Besides the controlled study that was conducted in the development phase, a larger randomized controlled trial (RCT) has subsequently been carried out with promising results (Balldin et al., 2019).

As part of the development of MAC, two models reflecting two different theoretical traditions were incorporated into the intervention. The first, Marte Meo (MM) was developed by Maria Aarts (2008) and may be considered normative and pedagogic, and the specified goal is to help parents (or other significant others) to identify ways in which they can support the development of the child for whom they are important. Central to the model is an idea of what constitutes supportive behaviour, and the principal method is the use of video analysis to identify examples

---

[1] Ingegerd Wirtberg died in February 2021. She was the driving force behind the development of MAC and the subsequent research projects. She is greatly missed by all who worked with her.

of such behaviour in the current interaction between significant adult and child and to see how they can be applied in different contexts.

It was decided from the start that it would be the school that initiated involvement in the project, and a referral would be accepted when it had the defined goal of supporting a specific child in his development so that his experience of school could become more positive. Since it was in the school that the behaviour of the child was first defined as being problematic, it was concluded that an intervention to support both the child and the teacher directly in the classroom where they worked together was the obvious starting point—reflecting the idea that it is often logical to try and solve problems in the context in which they emerge. To achieve a specific goal often requires specific resources and methods and it was felt that a normative, practical and pedagogic model such as MM would be an appropriate type of intervention to use in the school setting.

On the other hand, Coordination Meetings (CMs) reflect second-order cybernetic thinking, inspired by collaborative approaches such as *reflective processes* (Andersen, 1995), *language-systems* (Anderson, 1997) and *open dialogues* (Seikkula et al., 2003). CMs were created to provide a forum for significant adults (parents and teachers mostly) where they would be able to share their experience of the child. The coordinators' role was conceived of as a facilitator, who was to be responsible for establishing and maintaining a culture of epistemic trust, in which parallel and even conflicting narratives concerning the child could be shared and supported simultaneously. There is some resemblance here to the ideas about the "fifth province", a model created by McCarthy and Byrne (2008), in which a symbolic and safe place is created, where people can meet and engage in dialogical conversations.

The Systems Perspective

From the beginning, the team felt that adopting a systems perspective would be practical, as it easily accommodates different approaches. A systems perspective could allow the two separate interventions—MM and CMs—to be conceived of as two elements in a single, systemic intervention (MAC) (Axberg et al., 2021). Likewise, it would also help researchers and clinicians to maintain a high-level perspective from which they could think about both the internal workings of the two major social systems involved (school and family, but even others where relevant) as well as their relationships with each other.

Von Bertalanffy—the initial proponent of what he called a systems perspective or systems pedagogic—envisaged his approach as a meta-perspective that could help to relate specialized areas of research and knowledge in a coherent manner, thereby facilitating communication between experts (and laymen) (1972). As a philosopher of biology, he began the journey towards a systems perspective early in his career, and his first book after the acceptance of his doctoral thesis was entitled in English: *Modern Theories of Development: An Introduction to Theoretical Biology* (Oxford University Press; New York: Harper, 1933).

Parallel to Van Bertalanffy, Norbert Wiener (1948) developed a series of concepts that he called *cybernetics*. He was also fascinated by the organizational principles found in both living and mechanical systems, particularly in relation to the aspect of control. For example, how does a cell maintain a recognizable form and carry out those operations that are necessary for the maintenance of its own existence?

Wiener's cybernetics and Van Bertalanffy's general systems perspective are complementary: for example, a naturally occurring system (a flower, a cat) must be explored on its own terms if we wish to understand both how it is constructed and how it maintains its organization. On the other hand, an artificial system (a computer, a space probe) is consciously constructed using already understood principles and ideas that are chosen to enable them to fulfil the purpose their creators have in mind. To be able to understand how any complex system organizes and regulates itself, and use that understanding to support its functions (medicine and psychotherapy, for example, in the case of people; engineering in the case of mechanical systems), may involve many theories and techniques.

In a discussion of how he thinks that systemic psychotherapy has developed over the last few decades, Luigi Onnis (2016) talks about what he calls "the optics of complexity"—in which conceptualization in the field is influenced by our growing understanding of the nature of complex, dynamic systems. Also the chapters by de Flon and Sheenhan, and van Roosmalen in this volume give an illustration of this. Onnis further argues that such a perspective not only strengthens the challenge to the reductionism of classical physics as being the only valid scientific way of understanding or explaining the world, but does the same to any attempt to construct a holistic, "all-encompassing" perspective or theory. Onnis points out that the keyword in the paradigm of complexity is *plurality*. Every description of reality is limited and partial, even the systemic one. In practical terms, for example, the variety of human suffering requires a variety of approaches. This is something that Varela (1979) noted: the choice of different perspectives illuminates different aspects of whatever phenomenon is being studied: what is important is to be aware of the reason for the original choice, and how it influences the information generated.

A Brief Description of Marte Meo and Coordination Meetings

At the heart of MAC is a presupposition that when a child's behaviour is described by someone as being problematic (or positive, for that matter), then this description cannot be entirely understood as a simple representation some quality that is located within the individual child. Rather, any valuation of behaviour is produced in a network of interactions and relationships that exists between individuals in a specific context. Thinking in this way suggests that any possible intervention might benefit from trying to understand this network of relationships and encourage all parts of the network to collaborate with each other. The intervention described here is designed to both support the child and to strengthen the possibility of collaboration, and it consists of three separate parts or functions: Coordination Meetings (CMs), Marte Meo (MM) support in the pre-school/school—and, if the parents ask for it, Marte Meo support in the family (Wirtberg et al., 2013), as illustrated in Fig. 9.1. The core of this "collaboration model" is what has come to be known as *the working question*: "What is the need for developmental support for this child?" It is around this question that the entire intervention is focused.

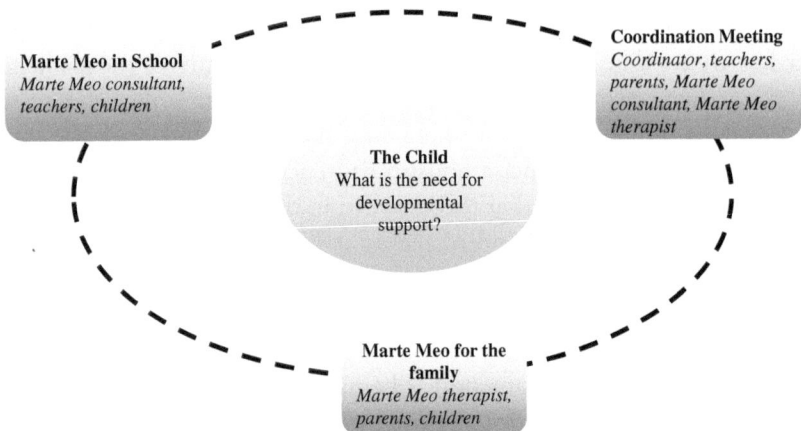

Fig. 9.1 An overview of the MAC model (*Source* Wirtberg et al. 2013, p. 18)

From the beginning, the team decided that the MAC workplace could be created where and when needed—there was no particular need to create a new department with their own offices. Instead, as qualified practitioners with the necessary skills were already in place in the county, albeit in different workplaces, it was decided together with the administrative and political leadership that when a referral was received a group with the necessary skills should quickly be assembled and a workspace allocated.

In Practice

The first coordination meeting takes place on a November evening in Sonny's school. The meeting includes both parents, the teacher who initiated the meeting and two of her colleagues, the Marte Meo guidance counsellor and the coordinator. The atmosphere is tense when the coordinator welcomes everyone and explains the purpose of the meeting. The father says he is in a hurry and the mother looks resigned. The teachers are also tense and everyone seems to be a little relieved when the coordinator takes clear control of the meeting. Everyone gets the opportunity to introduce themselves and after clarifying the purpose of the meeting, the coordinator describes how he intends to structure it. The reflective way of working is revealed when the coordinator starts to talk to the various participants in different groupings. Whoever is in the speaking position receives undivided attention and many follow-up questions. The coordinator is carefully trying to "tune in" and develop a supportive relationship with each person. The path to developing a relationship with trust is different for everyone, sometimes it is by talking football, sometimes by going straight to the "problem". When the teachers are asked what they are worried about, they talk about their efforts to help Sonny at school but how their attempts have had little effect. They are worried that the boy will "fall behind" in school and that he will continue "disrupting" the lessons. Their stories differ somewhat from each other and the coordinator tries to access their personal stories. The coordinator then turns to the parents and asks if there are things they recognize or don't recognize and if they want to comment on the teachers' stories. After this question, the conversation continues with the parents talking about their experiences, thoughts and feelings about Sonny and their relationship with him. The father shows more interest when he receives questions about himself, his work and his boy. The mother and the teachers look a little wary and suspicious when the father talks about his and the boy's common interests. The mother is tight-lipped and a little reserved when she is interviewed. She says that she thinks that the boy is doing well at home and that she thinks that they make too great demands on him at school and that he is also blamed for things that others have done. Finally, the coordinator gives the word to the Marte Meo guide and asks her to describe how she might be able to help. She explains concretely how she works and how by filming they will look at what Sonny needs for development support. The coordinator listens with interest to all meeting participants, asks follow-up questions, keeps order in the "listening" and "speaking positions" and then allows the various parties to reflect on each other's stories. The conversation climate changes slightly for the better as the meeting progresses, possibly the consequence of everyone being listened to with respect and interest, but perhaps also because the "conciliatory", curious and exploratory attitude adopted by the coordinator towards everyone is contagious. Experience has shown that often coordination meetings are initially marked by suspicion and latent conflicts, and this means that the coordinator must pay attention to actively working on a positive and conciliatory emotional attitude. The communication tools for this are humour, affirmation by using positive restatements, continually repeating back what someone has said to show that they have been heard, using every opportunity to make eye contact and having a warm tonality as often as possible. But above all by being genuinely interested in everybody's personal story.

In contrast to the Marte Meo intervention, the CMs in themselves have neither mandate nor function to achieve any specific change. Their primary purpose is to facilitate the communication between the school and the family by affirming the integrity of both. A second purpose is to ensure that the meetings always remain focused on their commission, or the purpose for which they have been created: what kinds of developmental support for the child seem to be required, and how can these ideas be applied in practice. Thus, the CMs tend to move between two domains: one that is more normative, in which monologic contributions from participants dominate, and during which work issues, goals and the Marte Meo effort are discussed. In the second domain, a more dialogic conversation is to be found, and here more individual and personal experiences and stories emerge. These are supported to exist side by side—and in this way, the possibility of new stories or "mutual creations" is made possible. Being a more personal, sharing conversation, this domain also tends to be less normative.

At the beginning of the development of the intervention, it was rather naively thought that the contents of the second domain were simply selected stories *that were about the child*. However, over time we became more aware that they were not just stories (both told and untold) about the child, but that they were also about the teller—the teachers and parents. The role of the coordinator is central to facilitate this shift of focus—from "the child" to "the child and me and us". This is helped by the fact that the coordinator comes from an "outside" position. Not being directly involved in either, she has no investment in either the school or the home and the work being carried out there, which helps her to remain neutral in relation to both systems, allowing her to be equally curious about and affirming of all participant's narratives concerning themselves and others. This position is also reminiscent of Boszormenyi-Nagy's idea of *multidirectional partiality* defined as being equally affirmative of all participants in the therapy process (Boszormenyi-Nagy & Krasner, 1986).

The coordinator has no other agenda than that of facilitating dialogical conversations. This she will do within the context of the meeting by listening, affirming and protecting the different narratives presented by both the school and the parents even when they are contradictory and conflicting. This is a challenging task, especially when the participants in the meeting are in conflict, but as systemic practitioners the coordinators are trained in how to be continually affirmative whilst remaining neutral by steadfastly remaining interested and curious in order to explore each and every speaker's intention and meaning. In this work, it was found that the use of reflective positions was very fruitful as it gives space for both inner and outer dialogues.

Being aware that the power relationship between school and family is reciprocal but not necessarily equal is important in this context, and becomes more important when conflicts are present. It makes it all the more important for the coordinator to strive to work in a way that is experienced as beneficial for all parts of the system. For example, early on in the developmental process we became deeply aware of the difference between *inviting* or *calling* people to a coordination meeting. If you seriously want people to come to a meeting and to be as "open" as possible, the participants need to feel right from the start that their thoughts, feelings, and experiences are genuinely important—that as prospective participants, they are important. Thinking in this way helps us to understand that invited participants should legitimately be able to influence when and where the meeting is to be held. A consequence of this approach is that it may be difficult to get the first meeting arranged, as there are often many different requests regarding time and place that must be accommodated and reconciled. However, over time, it became increasingly clear that this initial preparatory work—which could involve many telephone contacts and a lot of time—was of great importance for all that followed. It is well worth the effort to be thorough and respectful at this stage, even if it takes patience on the part of the coordinator to make an arrangement that works for everyone.

Another factor to be reckoned with is that some parents may have had their own difficulties in school or experienced that they were disadvantaged there by their former teachers—which might have an influence on their perception of the relationship with their child's present teacher, for example, by possibly feeling that they are inferior to or of lower social status than the teacher. At the same time, perhaps the teacher may feel themselves in a vulnerable and exposed position, liable to criticism and being questioned professionally by other staff in the school and by the school leaders, as well as by other children's parents. To establish epistemic trust, a safe context is necessary, so that the participants dare to expose themselves to the possible risks that personal statements might make them vulnerable to.

Another element that can help to make a meeting a safe place is to use of *contextual markers*: for example, clear information as to why the meeting has been called and who has called it, its structure, what its general purpose is, who is the leader, what are its specific goals, how the meeting will be run (rules) and what roles the participants have (Petitt, 2016). Another skill that helps is to be sensitive to what Øvreeide (1998) refers to as "identity markers", i.e. signals that are meant to inform others of how the individual perceives herself (and wishes to be perceived by others)—clues that reveal her social and individual identity. In the introductory "social phase" of the meeting, the coordinator will try and identify such markers and talk to the different participants about topics that contribute to their identity of competence or "adult identity". It can be about the relationship with the child, about school, but also if needed, about other areas of interest such as sports, work, cultural activity or (particularly in this area of Sweden) hunting.

The MM consultant has filmed a number of interactions between the teacher and Sonny. Some show structured contexts, such as when the teacher is giving instructions to the class, as well as unstructured situations, such as play. She analyses these short videoclips and then reviews them together with the teacher. In the previous review, the teacher observed that sometimes it seems as if Sonny might be signalling some kind of distress, but that the signals themselves are rather weak, and can easily be missed: for example, he drops his pen on the desk, or bends forward and leans his forehead on the desk. These signals have previously gone unnoticed by her since she has the whole class to attend to. Then, he bursts out in anger, but the teacher now concludes that it does not come "like a bolt from the blue", but happens after the distress signals that were neither seen nor responded to by anyone.

Together with the consultant she discusses how she can position herself differently in the classroom so that she can more easily see and so be able to respond to Sonny's signals. In the following review, the teacher and consultant see how, when the teacher has finished giving an instruction to the class, she notices Sonny dropping his pen on the desk. She goes over to him and bends down giving the opportunity to make eye contact and asks Sonny if he finds the task hard. He nods and mumbles that he can't solve it. She suggests that they can try together, and patiently she guides Sonny through the steps needed, and he succeeds in solving the task. Sonny and the teacher then look at each other with a radiant glow of happiness. The consultant suggests that they should show this videoclip in the next coordination meeting.

When they did so, Sonny's mother burst into tears. When asked about the meaning of her tears she said that she thought that Sonny and the teacher could not work together and that they didn't like each other, but here she can see how much they enjoy working together and how they really seem to like one another. Sonny's father had been silent up to this point, but then says that he also finds it difficult to read Sonny's signals at times and wonders if it is still possible for a Marte Meo therapist to come home and film him and Sonny, an offer that had been made to him earlier, but which he had declined.

Marte Meo makes extensive use of video feedback. The intervention begins with significant adult (e.g. a teacher or parent) identifying and defining the nature of a problem they have in relation to a child. This is done together with a Marte Meo consultant in the school or Marte Meo therapists in the home. Then they are asked to specify what they would like to achieve in that relationship. In the next step, a brief (5–10 minutes) interaction between the adult and child in the classroom/home is filmed by the MM consultant/therapist. The MM consultant/therapist then analyses and edits the film using the development-supporting principles that constitute the core theoretical concept in MM (from the perspective of the adult): (1) identifying the child's focus of attention; (2) confirmation of sharing focus; (3) waiting for the child's reaction—beginning of turn-taking; (4) naming experience; (5) taking responsibility for the development of turn-taking; (6) ongoing naming, structure and leadership; (7) triangulation; and (8) starting and ending signals.

In the next step, the edited film is reviewed together with the adult. This will normally result in the assigned of a specific homework for the adult which is to be tested in interaction with the child. The purpose is to identify the child's specific needs of developmental support and explore which responses from the adult seem to promote positive development. After that a new film of a brief interaction is recorded, analysed, and reviewed and together the MM consultant/therapist and adult explore if and how the task suggested in the homework has been of any benefit. If needed a new homework is assigned, new films are then made.

In Fig. 9.2, the MAC intervention is described step by step.

Final Reflexions

As noted earlier, Marte Meo is both normative and pedagogic in nature, and we have chosen to combine that method with a reflective working method that is grounded in a social constructionist theory and which is non-normative by definition. We have found that the two models work well in a complementary manner, as long as one is faithful to each model when using it or when discussing it—and do not confuse the two sets of concepts. This is again an example contextual markers: "Now we are applying Marte Meo, so we think and act from that theory and practice" or "Now we are applying CMs".

In considering and creating the structure for the coordination meetings, the coordinator obviously uses some normative ideas: for example, both theory and experience suggest that where possible it is generally beneficial if both parents are present (whilst always being sensitive to factors which make it inappropriate for them to be in the same room at the same time). Another is transparency: if relationships are to enjoy epistemic trust and mutual respect, again experience suggests that it is important that the leader of the meeting incorporate such principles into her own behaviour. A third—as we noted above—concerns the contextual markers that are used to structure and guide the meetings—and so

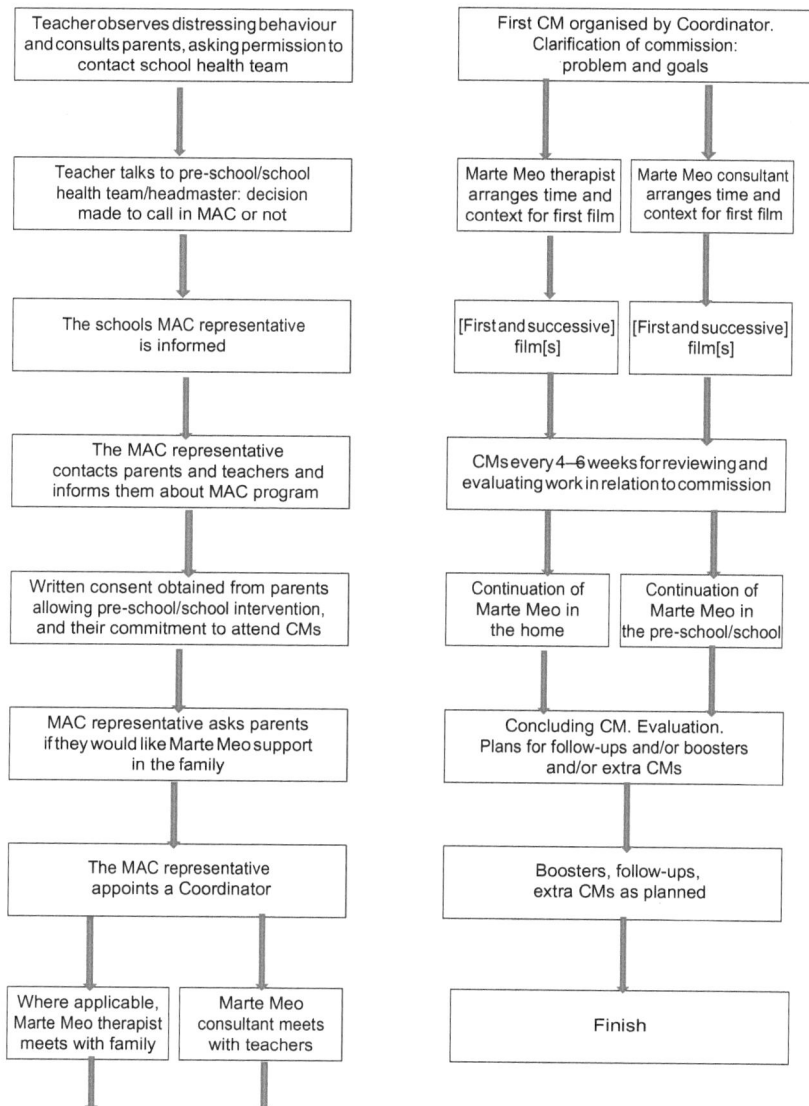

Fig. 9.2 Flowchart describing the MAC intervention (*Source* Wirtberg et al. 2013, p. 120)

on. However, once the meeting is under way, the coordinator switches to mainly working with a non-normative methodology based on collaborative and reflective principles. The coordinator is curious and exploratory, leading the process so that different opinions, thoughts and claims are allowed to coexist without demands for consensus, and where everyone has the right to speak and be listened to. Here, too, it is important to be "faithful to the model"; for example, the coordinator's credibility would immediately be destroyed if certain statements or opinions were given interpretive priority in the meeting. The only thing that participants need to agree to is the commission—the reason for the existence of the meetings. Since this is positively worded ("We are here to see how we can help the child develop in a positive way") and does not focus on the child as being a problem, it is normally easy to agree on that issue.

The division of models into the categories "normative" and "non-normative" is, of course, yet another construction of categories (see chapter by Axberg and Petitt in this volume) and it can be said of both of the models used in this intervention (and of all models in general), that they contain the possibility of both aspects. As was noted earlier, understanding is generated by the perspective chosen to look from. In practice, the open and reflective method is tightly controlled so that everyone gets their space to speak or listen and reflect on what they have heard. The clear management of the process provides the security and predictability that participants need to dare to speak freely, and to want to open up and to really listen to others. The Marte Meo model with its normative and relatively simple set of criteria designed to support children's development invites open reflection on the nature and meaning of interaction for both teachers and parents.

We cannot of course "know", but those who participated in the interventions became convinced that the combination of a more normative "hands on" intervention with a more non-normative intervention was beneficial. It is noteworthy that both studies mentioned here not only showed promising results in terms of effectiveness, but possibly the most interesting result was that there were few dropouts. In reviews of intervention studies concerning children displaying disruptive behaviour, the dropout rate is commonly as high as over 45% (Chacko et al., 2016; Lai et al., 1997). In the first controlled study, all teachers and all parents remained in the intervention and the follow-up study. In the second study, the RCT, all remained in the intervention, and only about 10% dropped out of the follow-up for various reasons. A further suggestion concerning the importance of the CMs is to be found in a qualitative study that explored parent's and teacher's experiences of them. Here, it was found that CMs seem to promote a non-blaming climate, giving room for different voices and opinions in a manner that strengthened the link between home and school (Tarnow Håkansson & Hansson, 2015).

References

Aarts, M. (2008). *Marie Meo: Basic manual* (2nd ed.). Aarts Production.

Andersen, T. (1995). Reflecting processes; acts of informing and forming: You can borrow my eyes, but you must not take them away from me! In S. Friedman (Ed.), *The reflecting team in action, collaborative practice in family therapy* (pp. 11–37). Guilford Press.

Anderson, H. (1997). *Conversation, language and possibilities: A postmodern approach to therapy*. Basic Books.

Aponte, H. J. (1976). The family-school interview: An eco-structural approach. *Family Process, 15*(3), 303–311. https://doi.org/10.1111/j.1545-5300.1976.00303.x

Axberg, U., Hansson, K., Broberg, A. G., & Wirtberg, I. (2006). The development of a systemic school-based intervention: Marte Meo and coordination meetings. *Family Process, 45*, 375–389.

Axberg, U., Petitt, B., & Wirtberg, I. (2021). Marte Meo and coordination meetings: A systemic, school-based intervention. In M. Mariotti, G. Saba, & P. Stratton (Eds.), *Handbook of systemic approaches to psychotherapy manuals. Integrating research, practice, and training*. Springer.

Balldin, S., Bergström, M., Wirtberg, I., & Axberg, U. (2019, November 21). Marte Meo and Coordination meetings (MAC): A systemic school-based video feedback intervention—A randomised controlled trial. *Child and Adolescent Social Work Journal, 36*, 537–548. https://doi.org/10.1007/s10560-018-0580-2

Boszormenyi-Nagy, I., & Krasner, B. R. (1986). *Between give and take: A clinical guide to contextual therapy* (ch. V). Routledge.

Chacko, A., Jensen, S. A., Lowry, L. S., Cornwell, M., Chimklis, A., Chan, E., Lee, D., & Pulgarin, B. (2016, September 01). Engagement in behavioral parent training: Review of the literature and implications for practice. *Clinical Child and Family Psychology Review, 19*(3), 204–215. https://doi.org/10.1007/s10567-016-0205-2

Lai, K. Y., Chan, T. S., Pang, A. H., & Wong, C. K. (1997). Dropping out from child psychiatric treatment: Reasons and outcome. *International Journal of Social Psychiatry, 43*(3), 223–229.

McCarthy, I. C., & Byrne, N. O. R. (2008). A fifth province approach to intracultural issues in an Irish context. In M. McGoldrick & K. Hardy (Eds.), *Revisioning family therapy: Race, class, culture and gender in clinical practice.* Guilford Press.

Onnis, L. (2016). From pragmatics to complexity: Developments and perspectives of systemic psychotherapy. In M. Borcsa & P. Stratton (Eds.), *Origins and originality in family therapy and systemic practice* (pp. 13–23). European Family Therapy Association Series. Springer. https://doi.org/10.1007/978-3-319-39061-1_2

Øvreeide, H. (1998). *Samtal med barn. Metodiska samtal med barn i svåra livssituationer* [Conversations with children. Methodical conversations with children in difficult life situations]. HøyskoleForlaget.

Petitt, B. (2016). *System, context and psychotherapy. Towards a unified approach.* CreateSpace Independent Publishing Platform.

Seikkula, J., Arnkil, T. E., & Eriksson, E. (2003). Postmodern society and social networks: Open and anticipation dialogues in network meetings. *Family Process, 42,* 185–203.

Talia, A., Duschinsky, R., Mazzarella, D., Hauschild, S., & Taubner, S. (2021). Epistemic trust and the emergence of conduct problems: Aggression in the service of communication. *Frontiers in Psychiatry, Sec. Child and Adolescent Psychiatry.* https://doi.org/10.3389/fpsyt.2021.710011

Tarnow Håkansson, P., & Hansson, A. (2015). *"Samordningssamtal, en ren lyx!" Föräldrars och pedagogers upplevelser av s amordnings samtal in om interventionsmodellen Marte Meo och Samordningssamtal* [Coordination Meetings, a pure luxury. Parents' and teachers' experience of Coordination Meetings in the Intervention "Marte Meo and Coordination Meetings (MAC)"]. Department of psychology, University of Gothenburg, Gothenburg.

Thayer, L. (1972). Communication systems. In E. Laszlo (Ed.), *The relevance of general systems theory: Papers presented to Ludvig von Bertalanaffy on his seventieth birthday* (pp. 93–122). Braziller.

Varela, F. J. (1979). *Principles of biological autonomy* (ch. 8–10). North Holland.

Von Bertalanffy, L. (1972). The history and status of general systems theory. *Academy of Management Journal, 15*(4), 407–426. https://doi.org/10.2307/255139

Wiener, N. (1948/1961). *Cybernetics: Or control and communication in the animal and the machine*, 2nd ed. MA: MIT Press.

Wirtberg, I., Petitt, B., & Axberg, U. (2013). *Mare Meo and coordination meetings: MAC. Cooperating to support children's development*. Palmkrons.

10

The Community Relations Model (CoRe): An Integrated Systems Response to Early Mental Health Support for Children and Families in Communities

Marc van Roosmalen

Mental health is contextual—both intimate and distal. Our realities are entangled with those of others, and so is our well-being—personal, emotional and social. Mental health is a political and societal issue that needs to be addressed by governments and society at all levels. The pandemic and social movements such as the Me Too and Black Lives Matter are ample evidence of the impact of isolation, discrimination and inequality on vast sections of society and their well-being. Mental health services, while still offering specialist therapeutic support for young people and families who struggle the most, need to be embedded within a broader systemic or ecologic service model addressing the broader causes of mental health problems. Studies of the incidence of child mental health problems across Europe, United States and the UK all identified a significant upward trend in prevalence over the last decade. In the UK, a review noted a rise in child mental health disorders from 1 in 9 in 2017

M. van Roosmalen (✉)
East London National Health Service Foundation Trust, London, UK
e-mail: marc.vanroosmalen@nhs.net

© The Author(s) 2024
S. M. Myra et al. (eds.), *New Horizons in Systemic Practice with Children and Families*, Palgrave Texts in Counselling and Psychotherapy,
https://doi.org/10.1007/978-3-031-38111-9_10

to 1 in 6 for 6–16-year-olds in 2020 (Children's Commissioner, 2021; House of Commons Health & Social Care Committee, 2021).

The Community Relations Model (CoRe) provides a new horizon for child mental health care—a framework for a relational and community model of mental health service for children and families (first published as a Systems Relations Model but since broadened to become an integrated systems model). It explains at what levels interventions need to be planned and delivered, and how. It is an evolving and aspirational model, going through constant iterations and learning cycles, while being open to criticism, as part of larger and more powerful systems and influences (van Roosmalen, 2018; van Roosmalen et al., 2013).

The Community Relations Model reconceptualizes a child mental health service, and how it can be operationalized, shifting from an overwhelmingly deficit or illness model of mental health to a relational, resilience-based and integrated systems model, with a focus on thriving communities and professional systems, rather than individuals. Publicly funded Child and Adolescent Mental Health Services (or, CAMHS) in the UK are structured to offer specialist mental health services to children and families predominantly by specialist therapeutic treatment, from early brief support for children and training for frontline staff such as in schools (through community-based teams where available) to specialist and highly specialist multi-disciplinary team provision and inpatient treatment. It is the common Western contemporary model. The broader causes and maintaining factors of mental health difficulties are considered rather than one that is symptom and thus, effect focused. In order to remedy the contextual causes of mental distress and ill health, a re-imagining of what constitutes mental health conceptually and building a service that starts to address these causes, operationally, is required. The concept of resilience is also re-considered.

The Community Relations (CoRe) Model—An Integrated Systems Response

.......he realizes that the truth is infinitely more complicated, that we are beautiful even as we are all part of the problem, and that to be part of the problem is to be human. (Doerr, 2022, p. 524)

The first step in re-thinking child mental health provision is to acknowledge that how current services are planned and delivered needs to be critically evaluated, particularly in the context of overwhelming demand and the lack of resources to respond adequately. Essentially, mental health services themselves are a crucial part of the change required.

The Community Relations Model is a continuation and broadening of the Systems Relations Model, explained by the author as consisting of a three function service model (van Roosmalen, 2018; van Roosmalen et al., 2013) that emerged from a study conducted with an early intervention schools and early years (0–5 years) CAMH service in the UK:

- Function 1: The offer of early specialist support to targeted children and families where children are struggling with their mental well-being.
- Function 2: A systemic function within the case work, where the CAMHS practitioner works with the systems interacting with the targeted children and families. This enables a collective and contextual understanding and formulation to be agreed around the problems experienced by the child, with a collective plan of support. The second function works across a four-phase case pathway. This function emerged from local research (van Roosmalen et al., 2013). This function has a particular focus on the first two phases of the case pathway, called the 'collaborative problem formulation' phases, where the network that interacts with the child in their everyday life collaborate on a plan of support with each other. The function is, however, applied across the phases of the pathway.

– Function 3: A universal intervention function. This contains whole school approaches, where the wider understanding of mental health is shared with schools, communities and other relevant stakeholders. It includes developing co-productive strategies and approaches to improve the well-being not only of individual children, but also the resilience and well-being of communities and agencies where children live and go to school and from whom they receive support. Examples are psycho-education strategies, and workshops for school staff to help them work with children with mental health vulnerabilities in order to keep them included in their education.

The first two functions are implemented by Child and Adolescent Mental Health Service practitioners within their early specialist casework with children and families, the school and other agency practitioners. They are not mutually exclusive functions, with the expertise of the CAMHS practitioner widening in their conceptualization of the inter-actional nature of mental health and distress. In this way, the child's mental health becomes 'everyone's business' (a term coined in the United Kingdom to try to engage all agencies in taking responsibility for children's mental health).

The principle across all three functional levels of practice is a rela-tional approach to working with children and their families and the multiple interacting systems they live within. For example, training for schools on mental health is not only symptom focused but explains how mental health difficulties arise from the living context and experiences of children, including within their schools.

The Community Relations Model, illustrated in Fig. 10.1, has evolved into a three-dimensional approach that explains:

1. Dimension 1: How resilient children and families develop in commu-nities, and factors that affect well-being.
2. Dimension 2: How frontline practitioners such as school staff can be resilient and support vulnerable children and families.

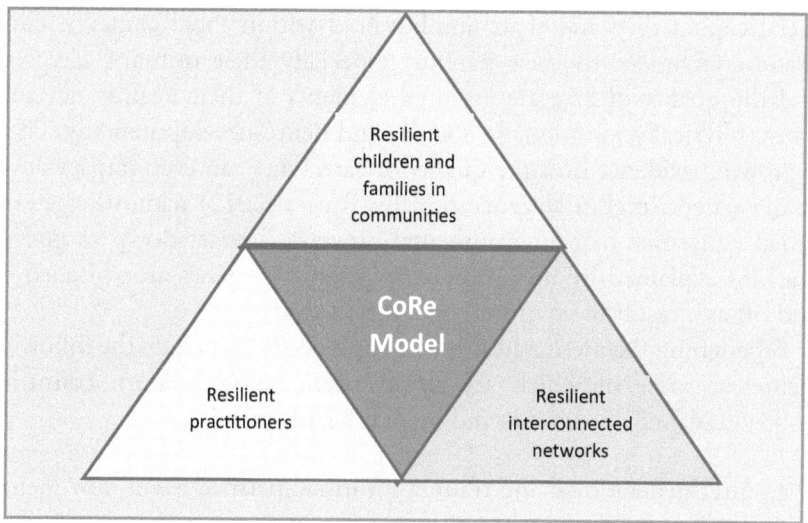

Fig. 10.1 The Community Relations Model (CoRe): developing resilient communities and professional networked systems working together

3. Dimension 3: How interconnected networks can work together—family, community and professional/agencies—to be resilient, reflective and where active learning and co-production of services is possible.

The model is a result of continuing cycles of service evaluation and research into the most effective and impactful ways of working with schools, early years' settings, Early Help social care services and communities.

CoRe Dimension 1: Resilient Children and Families Living in Communities

Children's development occurs within a context of proximal and distal factors impacting on them, through their parents and wider families, communities and broader groupings such as their ethnicity, and the social capital they and their families hold within these contexts. Children's attachment to their parents, especially their primary caregiver, and the quality of care are essential elements of their healthy development, physically, emotionally, socially and neuro-developmentally. There is growing evidence how the quality of caregiving can even impact down to the genetic level inter-generationally. Rutter (2012) acknowledged the broad consensus that environmental processes impact down to genetic level (as explained by the study of epigenetics)—genes are switched on and off as a result of environmental interactions.

Broadening the mental health construct needs to include the following elements, some of which are already permeating Western countries' policy guidance documents and mental health practice:

- an inter-generational and trauma-informed perspective of how mental well-being develops—that all strategies by parents, carers, children (and all stakeholders interacting with them, including practitioners) are adaptive strategies to survive and have their needs met as best they can. The growing discipline of epigenetics is discovering that the childhood experiences of parents can be transmitted to their children and then their grandchildren in a perpetuating cycle.
- Children and their families hold their unique inter-generational stories, and that requires CAMHS practitioners to contextually and systemically formulate in order to understand and work with the family.
- Adverse childhood experiences shape the way children and young people relate to others in their lives, and that these relationships are replicated within schools and interactions with other agencies.
- Resilience and mindfulness are inter-relational and dynamic concepts and cannot just be 'taught' to children didactically. Mindful and resilient communities will engender resilient children, not the reverse.
- Influences on mental health such as discrimination, poverty and lack of social capital need to be explicitly acknowledged. These experiences often occur across multiple generations as seen, for example, in the Black Lives Matter movement.

All of the above elements need to become part of the normal discourse about mental health, and a core part of training in mental health for all of those working in universal children's services, from schools, children's centres, child health, social care and other children-focused agencies. This will aid the emergence of sub-ordinate community narratives that have not been acknowledged, from narratives of failure (and blame) to an appreciation of the challenges that communities and families can face, as a first step to addressing the causes. In the author's experience, this leads to an enlivened dialogue about mental health and takes a significant step to demystifying, destigmatizing and normalizing mental health concerns.

Resilience and Inequality

In terms of re-evaluating the concept of resilience, longitudinal studies have shown that resilience is a dynamic process between the individual and their environment, both proximal and distal. It is a fluid interaction between the two over time (Rutter, 2012). Resilience is thus less an individual trait and more of a quality of the child's social and physical ecology (Ungar, 2011).

Faulconbridge et al. (2019) surmised from the research on the relational nature of resilience, that:

> …..if we take this wider evidence informed view that resilience is a dynamic interaction between the individual and their ecology, over time, it opens up exciting, and perhaps more helpful concepts of what a mental health intervention is and how we conceptualise mental health services. (p. 49)

The training needs to acknowledge the (distal) societal causal factors of mental health, as evidenced by extensive reviews conducted by Wilkinson and Pickett (2009, 2018). Through studying the social, health and mental health outcomes data of the wealthiest twenty nations in the world, a direct causal relationship was found to exist between social inequality and mental health:

Inequality affects the vast majority of the population, not only the poor minority.....larger income differences across a society immerse everyone more deeply in issues of status competition and insecurity. (Wilkinson & Pickett, 2018, p. 21)

These findings are essential in helping all stakeholders to understand and acknowledge the wide range of factors impacting on children's mental health, and that it is not a sign of their individual failure, or of their family, but that they are impacted by other wider influences. This would make it easier for communities and families to engage in dialogues about their children's, and their own, mental well-being.

Wilkinson and Pickett's findings are consistent across social, health and mental health outcomes:

It is because inequality affects most people that the differences in rates of health and social problems between more and less equal societies are often very large indeed. We found that mental illness and infant mortality rates were two to three times as high in more unequal countries. (Wilkinson & Pickett, 2018, p. 21)

CoRe 2: Resilient Frontline Practitioners Working with Children and Families

The second dimension addresses how frontline practitioners can develop and maintain their resilience and well-being while educating and supporting children and their families. Schools and other frontline agencies, such as children's centres, are increasingly seen as central points of contact for children and families and more emphasis is placed on schools to provide more holistic services rather than only education. School staff are increasingly faced with vulnerable children and families in their daily work, and there is broad acknowledgement that they require support and training in how to respond to this growing need.

Emotional Awareness and Responsive Practice

In order to develop their resilience, frontline practitioners would benefit from becoming more aware of their feelings and how to manage these in their relationships with others, particularly in an environment such as a school. This will enable them to be more mindful and compassionate towards themselves and others and to appreciate that all feelings and reactions are understandable (see Fig. 10.2), both theirs and those of the children. By accepting these feelings and understanding them (and crucially, having opportunities to do so) can lead to greater insight into both their own and the child and family's emotional worlds (see further Figs. 10.3 and 10.4) and thus supporting them at a universal level.

An example of an exercise with frontline practitioners is:

Can you think about a situation you have been in with a child:

– How did the child make you feel?
– Accept this feeling, what is its meaning for you?
– What might be replicated – for the child?
– What the meaning of the behaviour might be?
– How can you respond to the behaviour AND accept and validate the underlying meaning/need?

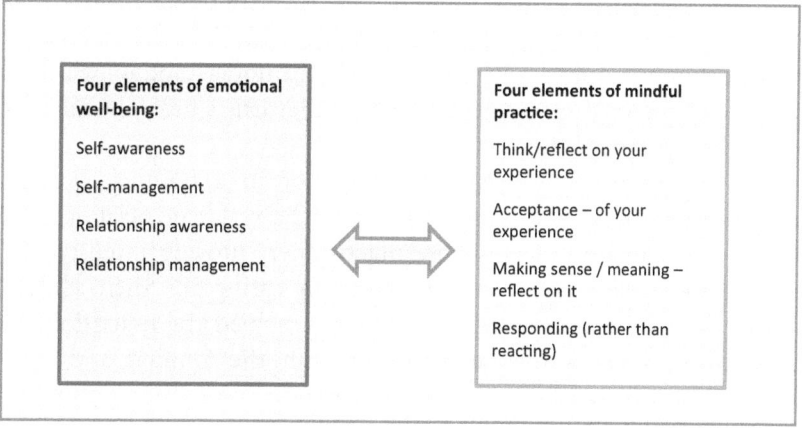

Fig. 10.2 The reflective practitioner: responsive and mindful practice

Actively supporting the increased emotional and relational awareness and resilience of frontline practitioners helps them to deal with the everyday stress they face in the current climate of the increasing amount and complexity of mental health, social and health needs of the communities they serve. It can also help prevent the cumulative emotional impact of these daily interactions on their mental well-being. Schools' staff are often the primary source of support that young people and their parents turn to when experiencing emotional distress. They need continuing support in how to manage it.

Interacting Stories of Practitioners with Children and Their Families

Practitioners can practise to become reflective about the stories and histories that children carry as well as how their own stories and histories inform their interactions with the children they work with. This will support a realization of how their own reality is interpreted through the lens of their own experiences and that this is also the case for others. They learn generally that this is what gets played out in relationships between people. Practitioners can benefit from using a reflective relational framework which can help them understand both the interactions between them and the families they support, and the emotional impact it can have on them as a result. As stated by Axberg and Petitt in their chapter in this volume, a child's behaviour can only be understood by within the network of interactions and relationships that exists between them and others in a specific context.

This framework was used by the author in a training workshop and continued reflective learning sets with Early Help social care children's service practitioners. These practitioners provide intensive early support to families who are struggling in caring for their children. The CoRe Model and reflective framework helped the practitioners to form strong collaborative relationships with the families and reduce their own stress in having to be the agent to solve the family's problems (van Roosmalen & Parrish, paper in preparation for submission). When reflecting on children's behaviour, practitioners can consider what emotions are being communicated, and what the underlying meaning of their emotions are. Behaviours are seen as compromised needs, and the challenge is, and was to understand the stories that are told through these. When faced with a vulnerable child's needs, the challenge would be how *to* connect with, not control, the child, which is often an issue school staff are faced with. Schools are environments where there are strict codes of behaviour, and where control is a big concern.

Figure 10.3 illustrates an interaction that regularly occurs between Early Help (Social Care Children's Services) staff and families, or teaching or other frontline staff, with a parent or child. In order for the practitioner to come to an understanding of the interaction, an exercise like the following can be used:

Think of a situation that has taken place with a student that has aroused a strong reaction in you. Think about your reaction, emotional and physical, and what it could say about:

You – your story and experiences
The parent + child – his/her stories and experiences
Something that is happening in the interaction between you

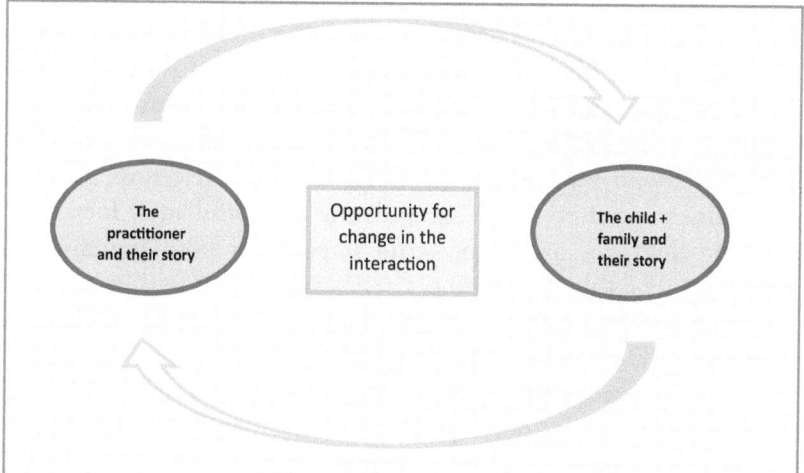

Fig. 10.3 The practitioner, the child and the family—interacting stories

Children and young people enter the school environment with estab-lished patterns of relating, and adaptive strategies from their families and communities that they replicate with school and other agency staff. Frontline practitioners often get drawn into these replicating patterns of relating, which can become toxic and a 'battle for control' can ensue, which can spiral out of control and lead to school exclusions and disengagement with education. With many children, minor school adjustments are possible, but many will not be able to make more signifi-cant adjustments, which can lead to frustrations on the part of the school and often, a resultant gradual polarization of positions taken by the child (and at times, the family) and school, leading to conflict and at times, a stalemate and exclusion.

The Reflective Relational Framework

The reflective relational framework (Fig. 10.4), in its simplest form of interacting stories (Fig. 10.3), illustrates how frontline practitioners who work with families, join the systems they are trying to support and become part of the interactional cycle with them. This is commonly described as the problem-determined system. This is an important shift from a linear pattern of thinking and practice, such as an objective outsider trying to effect change in the 'other' (child and/or family). Insight as to how this interaction occurs is necessary for frontline prac-titioners to understand how and why they get drawn into patterns of reactions and interaction. They can often go home after a day at school, for instance, with very powerful feelings of, anger, rejection, abandon-ment, sadness, or often, helplessness. Being a mindful adult for a young person or child can have a powerful impact, for both the child and practitioner. For this, developing a reflexivity of self within the inter-connecting systems of the school and family can ensure the resilience of the practitioner and benefit the child and family.

Frontline practitioners should be supported to learn how children's mental health problems develop (Dimension 1), and how they as prac-titioners can respond in a compassionate, mindful and reflexive way, as part of the system. They can learn how they are also part of

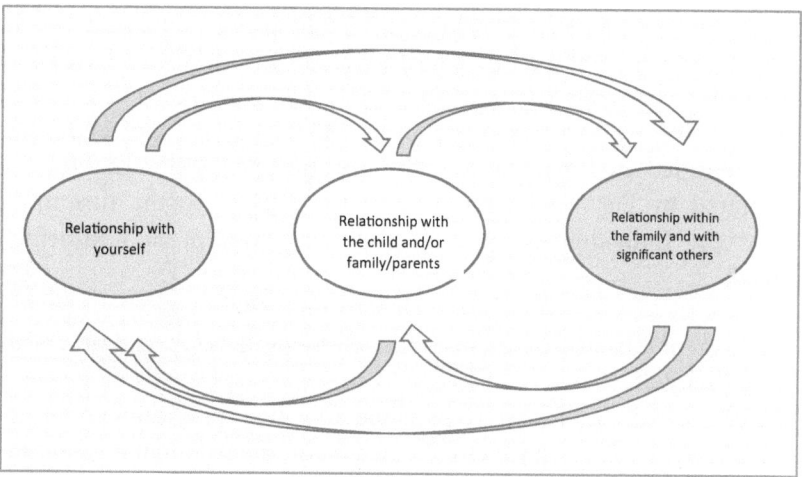

Fig. 10.4 The reflective relational framework

multiple systems that interact in particular ways (part of an organizational culture), cognizant of taking explicit positions of power ('there is something wrong with you and you need to change to fit in, otherwise you will become a failure'). This will develop their capacity to promote a relationship of more distributed power with families ("how can we work together to support your child who seems to be struggling", "we are struggling too with him/her", "we are at a loss and want to help"), validating the child's position (as an adaptive strategy) and that of the family (more of this in the third dimension).

CoRe 3: Resilient Interconnected Professional, Family and Community Systems

The third dimension describes how interconnected networks of practitioners, agencies, families and communities communicate and work together to meet the needs of vulnerable children and young people. A research study by the author and colleagues analysed how such interconnected systems can work. It identified the factors that improved the chances of constructive networking and led to positive outcomes for children in their mental health, educational inclusion, and improved the relationships between families and schools (van Roosmalen et al., 2013).

Partnership work between the local CAMH Service and school partners identified two distinct ways interconnected systems can function (illustrated by Fig. 10.5) (van Roosmalen, 2018). In the first model, coined the Individual Model, the following concept of well-being is applied:

- That mental health problems and well-being develop and are located in individuals.
- Children will often feel responsible for their predicament, as it is described as their 'problem', which can understandably lead to a defensive reaction.
- It is often the case in discourses of blame, that the most vulnerable in the system who has the least power, carries the most responsibility. This can be replicated in it also being a parent in social care discourses of responsibility ("they are a poor mother and failing").

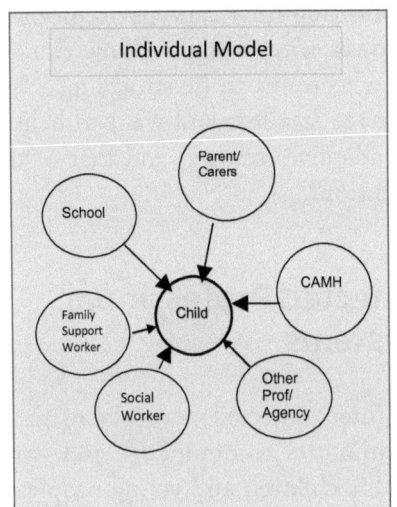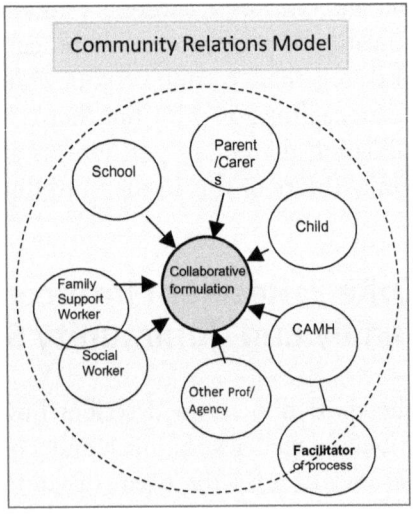

Fig. 10.5 Two models of interconnected systems working

- The system is helpless as the child or parent (or another) is the one who needs to change, and the system is trying to help them to change. This can disable a system, causing 'stuck systems' as they have failed to convince the family (of the need) to change.
- Responsibility, or its negative counterpart, blame, can be mirrored throughout the multi-agency system—such as the school seen to be failing the child pastorally, CAMHS not offering the therapy that is required for the child, all of which is contradictory to collaborative working.
- Different perspectives are often a source of conflict, with some views being valued over others, while others might be silenced in order to resolve the conflict in the system.
- The sum of the multi-agency network is less than its parts—which can lead to a 'stuck' and a demotivated system.

In the second model, originally named a Systems Relations Model (since updated to the Community Relations Model), the approach taken to mental health and well-being is:

- Mental health well-being and problems develop in relationships.
- No-one has sole responsibility and thus no one is blamed for the "problem" or to change—this leads to a lack of defensiveness, and where collaboration and dialogue are possible between stakeholders. It is acknowledged that everyone is part of the problem-determined system.
- Everyone involved in the child's life carries some responsibility, as all are relating with the child and all are part of a potentially resilient interconnected system.
- People in the system are empowered to change and support, which can be "enabling", as power and the capacity to change is distributed through the network.
- This encourages a culture of working together and collective responsibility.
- Differences between stakeholders, and multiple perspectives, are regarded as sources of richness and all views are valid and valued, increasing social capital.

— The sum of stakeholders becomes more than its separate parts, as it allows a greater pool of thinking and solutions and a motivated and energised professional and family network.

Schools form a key part of frontline systems providing universal and targeted support to children and young people. In terms of the context within which schools function, they evolve or adapt in connection with their neighbouring and community systems, and may show unpredictable patterns of cause and effect. Without a clear and strong self-organizing principle (and one that is reflective and thoughtful) schools can act and organize in similar ways as the communities they serve. Menzies Lyth (1960) described how organizations develop customs or patterns (which she described as defences) that have the effect of reducing anxiety, doubt or distress for staff. Child mental health service staff can act and react in similar ways, and also need to put themselves under the spotlight as part of the system that needs to look at its own culture and the defences it might have developed that might inhibit change.

De-polarizing the views between different stakeholders, such as school and the family, and the building of a collective understanding and formulation with the child, family and the school can lead to commonly agreed resolutions (Campbell & Groenbaeck, 2006). This exemplifies the second function of the model. Parents and school can often fall into positions of mutual blame, which can inhibit collaborative working and put more pressure on the child, a pattern also identified by Axberg and Pettit in their chapter in this volume. Using this function more broadly in relationships with other practitioners and agencies, and not only with specific children and families can lead to a culture of collaborative practice across stakeholders and more distributed power (van Roosmalen, 2018).

An Integrated Schools, Family and CAMHS Case Pathway

Figure 10.6 illustrates how both the first and second functions can work within a case pathway of a child. The pathway usually starts when the school discusses a child with a CAMHS practitioner due to their concerns for their mental health. All involved with the child at school form part of this consultation. The CAMHS practitioner then invites all professional and familial stakeholders to contribute to a dialogue about the difficulties the child is experiencing and their views, moving towards a systems-agreed collaborative formulation, using the principles of the CoRe Model described above. Collaboratively agreed support interventions are agreed to resolve the challenges being faced by all stakeholders. There is a focus on developing a collaborative formulation of the difficulties in the first two phases with the school, the family and any significant others involved, to process what can initially be divergent views. This requires attention and active facilitation, described by Axberg and Petitt in their chapter in this volume as establishing epistemic trust when variant and even conflicting narratives are held. The establishment of trust is required before a coherent plan of intervention can be agreed, laying the basis for collaborative and coordinated interventions. Phases 3 and 4 describe, respectively, the intervention and review phases, after which further intervention or closure is agreed. A more detailed explanation of the case pathway and the functional model is offered in van Roosmalen (2018). In a small-scale outcome study of school and parental views of this approach, family and school relationships were found to have improved (van Roosmalen & Gardner, 2007).

Wider Systems and Community-Based Resilience

In order to create systems and community-wide resilience and not only for individual targeted children and their systems, Faulconbridge et al. (2019) adapted Friedl and Carlin's (2009) recommendations (which were substantiated by longitudinal studies):

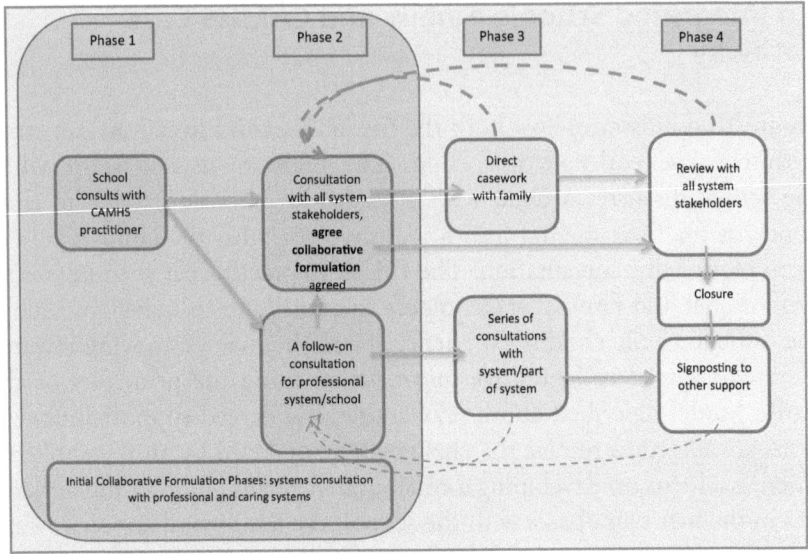

Fig. 10.6 A case pathway illustrating Function 1 and 2 of the CoRe Model

- Strengthen social relationships and community connections for children, young people and families.
- Enable and build social capital, social networks and social support within and between communities.
- Strengthen and repair relationships between communities and health and social care agencies, for example, enhancing community control by co-production.
- Improve the quality of the social relationships of care between children, young people and families, and professionals.

The above can potentially form part of universal school and community approaches in addition to being a crucial element of casework pathways when supporting targeted children and their families.

For example, local Early Help Children's Service practitioners (Social Care) were provided an introductory training to the Community Relations Model, which was followed by six months of group-based reflective learning sets. At these sets, they discussed current casework, integrated learning into practice, and were able to learn more widely in applying a wide range of systemic, resilience (and trauma-informed) techniques and practices into their daily practice. As a key aim of children's social care practice is to support more constructive parenting, this can easily be perceived by parents as blaming of them, for being a poor or failing parent. Early Help practitioners found that in order to break this interactional pattern they introduced the co-production of a three-generation genogram with the parents (and at times also with the children), a key technique learnt in the training. They discovered that it opened up a discussion about the parents' experiences of being parented themselves, which developed curiosity about their intentions as parents themselves, trans-generationally. The practitioners both led and enabled a conversation of appreciation of the difficult lives and circumstances of the families, resulting in a less defensive initial assessment phase with the families (van Roosmalen & Parrish, paper in preparation for submission). Linked to this was a key question they asked of their families, "What happened to you?" rather than a question such as "what is going wrong", the latter of which targeted deficits with the family, parent or child. This approach improved the relationships between their service staff and families.

Health Inequalities and Co-producing Services with Communities

One of the newly established local schools-based teams, who are part of a broader community-based early intervention mental health services for children and families (in the south of the UK of which the author is the lead), is working with 14 schools within an ethnically diverse and socially disadvantaged community to improve health equalities. They have embarked on a programme of engagement, planning and service delivery with all community stakeholders, including citizen stakeholders, community leaders, schools, local agencies and charities. The intention is to co-produce a needs-based integrated services response to mental health inequalities in the locality. A structured quality improvement methodology is being applied to encapsulate a broad response from all stakeholders that addresses contextual factors that have been identified as impacting on the mental health of the community. A broad theory of change and action plan is being co-produced with the wide range of stakeholders to produce an integrated multi-systems response to the community's needs.

Training for CAMHS Practitioners and the Dissemination of CoRe

For CAMHS community practitioners to feel competent and skilled to deliver the CoRe Model of practice, a systemic consultation training was designed and delivered following the study of the case pathway and three functional model (van Roosmalen et al., 2013). A qualitative study exploring the impact of the training on CAMHS practitioners' practice and confidence found the training to have greatly enhanced their skills in working with interconnected systems, fostering dialogue with at times stressed and overwrought schools systems, and improving their effectiveness in producing positive mental health outcomes (van Roosmalen et al., paper in preparation for submission). Gardner-Elahi's (2011) study of the impact of the style of consultation on school staff and parental consultees found the consultations had an empowering effect on them, and increased their confidence and competence to work together to support the children's needs.

The current schools teams have grown over the last few years following several years of recession and resultant public sector cuts in the locality of the author. They have an overview of the CoRe Model, but its application is variable and not yet systems wide. Aspects of the model are in the process of being applied to inform broader learning. The wider integrated systems model is now being applied and seen as the new horizon for local CAMH Services particularly in early support and community working. There is a current push for all mental health training to follow the CoRe approach, and to identify school practitioners who work daily with the most vulnerable children, to be trained in Dimension 2, which would follow a similar model of training to the Early Help training described earlier.

Conclusion—Why Is This Response so Urgent Now?

Studies on the incidence of child mental health problems across high-income countries (Barican et al., 2022), the United States (Whitney & Peterson, 2018), Europe (Neufeld, 2022; United Nations Children's Fund, 2021) and the United Kingdom (Children's Commissioner, 2021; House of Commons Health & Social Care Committee, 2021; Loades et al., 2020) have all identified a significant upward trend in prevalence in child mental health problems over the last decade. All studies internationally reveal the pandemic's further negative impact on children's mental health across all regions. Growing inequalities in countries such as the United Kingdom are only worsening its prevalence.

The social (including social media), environmental and economic factors impacting on children's mental health is almost universally acknowledged, yet the question remains why services are still only treating the effects being created by these proximal and distal causal factors, rather than starting to remodel and re-imagine child mental health services to start targeting the causes. The local effort, and that of the Community Relations integrated systems approach, is an attempt at targeting the factors impacting on mental health and developing community resilience. These innovations will need to be financially sustained long enough for them to evidence their effectiveness, as emphasized by Hannah (2010) in her paper on a sustainable future of an overstretched UK National Health Service.

We can be reassured by the existence of a wider than traditional evidence base. Quantum theory has grown in prominence as one of the dominant scientific theories explaining the physical world. Rovelli (2020) describes quantum theory as putting aside a reality which is object driven but in essence relational. Objects or things in the physical world exist in a context and not of themselves, with interaction an inextricable part of a phenomenon. This is expressed by the concept of contextuality:

We cannot separate out the properties of the objects from the objects interacting with them in order for these properties to be manifested in the first place. All of the (variable) properties of an object, in the final analysis, are such and exist only with respect to other objects. (Rovelli, 2020, p. 120)

All information we have about the world are of these correlations. The multiplicity of perspectives is, however, made coherent by a consistency where we influence (each other in) the way we 'see' the world. Rovelli says it is this consistency, called inter-subjectivity, which is the basis of our communal vision of the world. Public child mental health services need to change their horizon according to the emerging acknowledgement that 'the world' is impacting on children's mental health, and our services need to respond effectively to the causes, not only treat its effects. The latter would merely give responsibility, and its negative counterpart, blame, to children for their mental health problems, and that they need fixing, not the world around them.

References

Barican, J., Yung, D., Schwartz, C., Zheng, Y., Georgiades, K., & Waddell, C. (2022). Prevalence of childhood mental disorders in high income countries: A systematic review and meta-analysis to inform policymaking. *Evidence Based Mental Health, 25*, 36–44.

Campbell, D., & Groenbaeck, M. (2006). *Taking positions in the organisation.* Routledge.

Children's Commissioner. (2021). *The state of children's mental health services 2020/2021.* Children's Commissioner for England.

Doerr, A. (2022). *Cloud cuckoo land.* Fourth Estate.

Faulconbridge, J., Hunt, K., & Laffan, A. (2019). *Improving the psychological wellbeing of children and young people: Effective prevention and early intervention across health.* Jessica Kingsley Publishers.

Friedl, L., & Carlin, M. (2009). *Resilient relationships in the North West. What can the public sector contribute?* NHS North West and the Department of Health.

Gardner-Elahi, C. (2011). *Developing a model of consultees' understanding of mental health consultation in a school setting* (Unpublished doctoral dissertation). University of East London.

Hannah, M. (2010). *Costing an arm and a leg: A plea for radical thinking to halt the decline and the eventual collapse of the NHS.* International Futures Forum.

House of Commons Health and Social Care Committee. (2021). *Children and young people's mental health.* House of Commons HC17.

Loades, M. E., Chatburn, E., Higson-Sweeney, N., Reynolds, S., Shafran, R., Brigden, A., & Crawley, E. (2020). Rapid systematic review: The impact of social isolation and loneliness on the mental health of children and adolescents in the context of COVID-19. *Journal of the American Academy of Child & Adolescent Psychiatry, 59*(11), 1218–1239.

Menzies Lyth, I. (1960). A case-study in the functioning of social systems as a defence against anxiety. *Human Relations, 3*(2), 95–121.

Neufeld, S. (2022). The burden of young people's mental health conditions in Europe: No cause for complacency. *The Lancet Regional Health—Europe, 16,* 100364.

Rovelli, C. (2020). *Helgoland.* Allen Lane.

Rutter, M. (2012). Resilience as a dynamic concept. *Development and Psychopathology, 24*(02), 335–344.

Ungar, M. (2011). The social ecology of resilience: Addressing contextual and cultural ambiguity of a nascent construct. *American Journal of Orthopsychiatry, 81*(1), 1–17.

United Nations Children's Fund (UNICEF). (2021). *On my mind: The state of the world's children. Promoting, protecting and caring for children's mental health* (Regional Brief – European). UNICEF.

van Roosmalen, M. (2018). *A whole systems model of early intervention with schools and other frontline partner agencies: A systems relations approach.* In A. Vetere & E. Dowling (Eds.), *Narrative therapies with children and their families* (2nd ed.). Routledge.

van Roosmalen, M., Daniels, M., & Lawrence, H. (paper under peer review). *Clarifying a model for consultation: The impact of a consultation training on a CAMH Schools' service practice.*

van Roosmalen, M., & Gardner, C. (2007). *Key findings report: CAMH community services to education, Luton (Behaviour improvement programme and on track).* Unpublished report.

van Roosmalen, M., Gardner-Elahi, C., & Day, C. (2013). A systems-relations model for Tier 2 early intervention services with schools: An explorative study. *Clinical Child Psychology and Psychiatry, 18*(1), 25–43.

van Roosmalen, M., & Parrish, M. (paper in preparation for submission). *The impact of a relational training and practice approach on the everyday practice of early help social care practitioners supporting vulnerable families.*

Whitney, D. G., & Peterson, M. D. (2018). US national and state-level prevalence of mental health disorders and disparities of mental health care use in children. *Journal of the American Medical Association, Pediatrics, 173*(4) (April 2019), 389–391.

Wilkinson, R., & Picket, K. (2009). *The spirit level: Why more equal societies almost always do better.* Penguin.

Wilkinson, R., & Pickett, K. (2018). *The inner level: How more equal societies reduce stress, restore sanity and improve everyone's well-being.* Penguin.

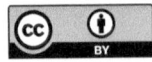

11

Epilogue

Siv Merete Myra, Tone Grøver, and Ulf Axberg

When we started working on this book, many countries in the world were still in lockdown because of the COVID-19 pandemic, including the countries of the authors. Lockdowns had lasted for almost two years, and our daily lives had gone through changes we could not have imagined before the pandemic. We developed new vocabularies and new ways of relating. And we had a clear feeling of how unpredictable and vulnerable life is and can be. At the same time, there continue to be so many other uncertainties, like the effects of climate changes, natural disasters, the destabilization of democracies, uncertain economic futures for many,

S. M. Myra (✉) · T. Grøver · U. Axberg
Department of Family Therapy and Systemic Practice, Faculty of Social Studies, VID Specialized University, Oslo, Norway
e-mail: siv.merete.myra@vid.no

T. Grøver
e-mail: Tone.Grover@vid.no

U. Axberg
e-mail: ulf.axberg@vid.no

migration, refugee flows, invasions and wars. We clearly feel how dependent we are on each other, as well as how difficult this interdependence can be.

In times of uncertainty, we are so fortunate to meet and work together with children and families. It can be both complex and challenging as well as rewarding work. We asked the authors, how can we use our systemic thinking and our systemic ways of working together with children and families in these times? The authors describe their different ways of meeting with children and families, who struggle with challenges, in their various contexts. But also, we asked the authors, how can systemic perspectives be beneficial in the exploration of openings, together with the children, their families and the professional practitioners around them. In particular, openings that can provide support in how to navigate in these circumstances and even make new possibilities become visible. The authors describe and reflect on how systemic approaches can be useful for practitioners: to safeguard children's rights through parental separation and divorce; in the conversations with families experiencing anticipatory grief; in meetings with parents struggling with substance use problems; in the exploration of feelings and experiences of children and youth and their families when experiencing gender incongruence; when working together with young people suffering from an eating disorder and their families; in relation to the psychiatric diagnosis of children; in working in families with children with disabilities; with school consultations; and how the school may be a possible context to provide early mental health community support for children and their families.

When we invited the authors to write a chapter their choice of theme was open, but we wanted them, all experienced practitioners, to share their experiences of the utility of a systemic approach to practice in various contexts. For example, how they in their practice had been inspired by what they had learnt from training, reading and research, but foremost, what they had learned and continued to learn in the conversations with children and families they had met. Perhaps, in light of the influences in systemic practice during these last decades, we should not be surprised that an overwhelming common thread in the contributions pointed to the need of finding ways, within an overarching systemic framework, to integrate perspectives from different traditions, even ones that might seem to be contradictory. They also highlighted the importance of and utility of bringing systemic perspectives into settings where other perspectives continue to dominate, and how multiple descriptions and what seem to be small shifts in perspective can make a great difference.

Much has been written about systemically informed work with children and families, so our wish for this book was to shed light over possible new horizons, and to expand what they can mean in our time. We hope that our priorities can bring forward new points of view within a large and important field of practice. We hope that this book can be a source of inspiration, as our common desire here was to keep the systemic field in motion, and to show how working together with children and families is such a privilege.

Index

© The Editor(s) (if applicable) and The Author(s) 2024
S. M. Myra et al. (eds.), *New Horizons in Systemic Practice with Children and Families*, Palgrave Texts in Counselling and Psychotherapy,
https://doi.org/10.1007/978-3-031-38111-9